T0136482

E.N.T.
MADE EASY

E.N.T.
MADE EASY

LINDA S. MACCONNELL
PA–C, MAEd, MPAS
Assistant Professor, Department of PA Studies,
AT Still University, Mesa, Arizona, USA
Advanced Practice Clinician, Enticare ENT,
Chandler, Arizona, USA

AMTUL SALAM SAMI
MBBS, BSc, ODTC, MCPS, MA, MSc
Specialist in E.N.T. and Allergy
Lewisham and Greenwich NHS Trust, London, UK

Scion

This is an Americanized and updated version of *ENT Made Easy* published by Scion Publishing Ltd in 2017 (ISBN 9781911510055)

© **Scion Publishing Ltd, 2019**
ISBN 9781911510307
First published 2019
All rights reserved. No part of this book may be reproduced or transmitted, in any form or by any means, without permission.
A CIP catalog record for this book is available from the British Library.

Scion Publishing Limited
The Old Hayloft, Vantage Business Park, Bloxham Road, Banbury OX16 9UX, UK
www.scionpublishing.com

Important Note from the Publisher
The information contained within this book was obtained by Scion Publishing Ltd from sources believed by us to be reliable. However, while every effort has been made to ensure its accuracy, no responsibility for loss or injury whatsoever occasioned to any person acting or refraining from action as a result of information contained herein can be accepted by the authors or publishers.

Readers are reminded that medicine is a constantly evolving science and while the authors and publishers have ensured that all dosages, applications and practices are based on current indications, there may be specific practices which differ between communities. You should always follow the guidelines laid down by the manufacturers of specific products and the relevant authorities in the country in which you are practicing.

Although every effort has been made to ensure that all owners of copyright material have been acknowledged in this publication, we would be pleased to acknowledge in subsequent reprints or editions any omissions brought to our attention.

Registered names, trademarks, etc. used in this book, even when not marked as such, are not to be considered unprotected by law.

Typeset by Medlar Publishing Solutions Pvt Ltd, India
Printed in the UK by 4edge Limited
Last digit is the print number 10 9 8 7 6 5 4 3 2 1

Contents

Preface ix

Acknowledgements x

Abbreviations xi

How to use this book xiii

Chapter 1   Clinical assessment 1

1.1   How to take a focused history of the ear, nose, and throat 2

1.2   How to perform a clinical examination of the ear,
         nose, and throat 4

1.3   Investigations in ENT 7

1.4   ENT tests performed during the clinical examination 8

1.5   Specialist tests 10

1.6   Vestibular function tests 15

1.7   Other investigations used in ENT 17

Chapter 2   Ear **19**

2.1   Basic anatomy of the ear 20

2.2   Differential diagnosis of ear problems 23

2.3   Deafness and hearing loss 25

2.4   Sudden hearing loss 28

2.5   Wax 30

2.6   Otitis externa 31

2.7   Otitis media 33

2.8   Cholesteatoma 36

2.9   Perforation of the tympanic membrane 38

2.10	Otosclerosis	40
2.11	Acoustic neuroma	43
2.12	The draining ear	45
2.13	Earache	47
2.14	Vertigo and dizziness	49
2.15	Benign paroxysmal positional vertigo	51
2.16	Labyrinthitis	53
2.17	Ménière's disease	55
2.18	Tinnitus	58
2.19	Presbycusis	60
2.20	Facial paralysis	61
2.21	Foreign body in the ear	65
2.22	Furuncle in the external auditory canal	66
Chapter 3	**Nose**	**67**
3.1	Basic anatomy of the nose and sinuses	68
3.2	Differential diagnosis of nose problems	71
3.3	Rhinitis	72
3.4	Epistaxis	77
3.5	Sinusitis	80
3.6	Fracture of the nasal bone	83
3.7	Anosmia	85
3.8	Foreign body in the nose	88
3.9	Furuncle in the nose	89
3.10	Perforation of the nasal septum	90
3.11	Sleep apnea	92
Chapter 4	**Throat**	**95**
4.1	Basic anatomy of the throat	96
4.2	Differential diagnosis of throat problems	98
4.3	Dysphagia	100
4.4	Tonsillitis	103
4.5	Peritonsillar abscess	106
4.6	Pharyngitis	107
4.7	A change in voice	109

4.8	Laryngitis	112
4.9	Stridor	114
4.10	Acute epiglottitis	118
4.11	Aphthous ulcer	120
4.12	Salivary gland stones	121
4.13	Foreign body in the throat	123
4.14	Halitosis	124
4.15	Neck mass	126
Chapter 5	**Pediatric ENT**	**129**
5.1	Introduction	130
5.2	Guide to ENT issues covered elsewhere	131
5.3	Pediatric history taking	132
5.4	Rhinitis	135
5.5	Sinusitis	136
5.6	Epistaxis	138
5.7	Nasal trauma	140
5.8	Obstructive sleep apnea	141
5.9	Adenoiditis	143
5.10	Cystic fibrosis	144
5.11	Hearing loss and deafness	145
5.12	Acute otitis media	147
5.13	Tinnitus	149
5.14	Vertigo	150
5.15	Laryngeal papillomatosis	152
Chapter 6	**Systemic disease affecting ears, nose, and throat**	**153**
6.1	Introduction	154
6.2	Skin disorders	154
6.3	Eye diseases	154
6.4	Nervous system and neurological diseases	155
6.5	Endocrine diseases	155
6.6	Congenital disorders	155
6.7	Vascular disease	155
6.8	Maxillofacial diseases	156

6.9   Bone and joint pathology 156

6.10   Gastroenterology 156

6.11   Medication 156

Chapter 7   Key operations in ENT **157**

Index 161

Preface

This book is a "translation" from English to language more commonly used in the United States. This edition of the book therefore removes the slight distraction which may be provided by reading English vernacular instead of US vernacular language.

Disorders of the ears, nose, and throat and their related symptoms are some of the most common presenting concerns in primary care. While many may be managed in primary care, some may require referral to an otolaryngology clinic.

Evaluation and treatment of ENT disorders is best managed by remembering the similarities and co-dependence of each of the systems. Clinicians will find this book to be of assistance in understanding the anatomy and physiology of ENT.

The book is helpful for clinicians because it provides necessary information in terms of clinical presentations, diagnostics, and management of conditions and their complications for patients of all ages, from pediatrics to geriatrics.

Chapter 6 of this book describes systemic diseases affecting the ears, nose and throat/larynx. This may represent the presenting concerns the patient has, leading to the diagnosis of systemic disease, and so providing a good review for clinicians of many specialties.

ENT Made Easy is a concise guide which provides a connection between theoretical knowledge and clinical practice, with all the basics needed to care for common ear, nose, and throat diseases in a variety of clinical situations.

Linda S. MacConnell, PA-C
January 2019

Acknowledgements

I would like to thank Dr Amtul Salam Sami (and her daughter Dr Nida Ahmed who contributed one of the chapters) for allowing me to Americanize her book.

Abbreviations

ABR	Auditory brainstem response
ACE	Angiotensin-converting enzyme
ANA	Antinuclear antibody
ANCA	Antineutrophil cytoplasmic antibodies
BPPV	Benign paroxysmal positional vertigo
C&S	Culture and sensitivity
CBC	Complete blood count
CMP	Complete metabolic panel
CPAP	Continuous positive airway pressure
CRP	C-reactive protein
CSF	Cerebrospinal fluid
CT	Computerized tomography
EAC	External auditory canal
ECG	Electrocardiogram
ED	Emergency Department
EEG	Electroencephalogram
ENG	Electronystagmography
ENT	Ear, nose, and throat
ESR	Erythrocyte sedimentation rate
FESS	Functional endoscopic sinus surgery
FNA	Fine needle aspiration
GERD	Gastroesophageal reflux disease
GI	Gastrointestinal
IAC	Internal auditory canal
INR	International normalized ratio
LFT	Liver function test
MDT	Multidisciplinary team
MRI	Magnetic resonance imaging
NSAID	Non-steroidal anti-inflammatory drug
OAE	Otoacoustic emissions

OM	Otitis media
OSA	Obstructive sleep apnea
PPI	Proton pump inhibitor
RAST	Radioallergosorbent test
TB	Tuberculosis
TFT	Thyroid function test
TMJ	Temporomandibular joint
U&Es	Urea and electrolytes
USS	Ultrasound scan
VNG	Videonystagmography

How to use this book

Conditions affecting the ear, nose, or throat are common in clinical practice and reduce quality of life. This book is your companion and guide to approaching and managing the symptoms of ENT diseases.

The book begins with the basic principles and methods of carrying out an effective **clinical assessment** and explains, in detail, the investigations which are key to exploring these conditions. Importantly, the book is patient-centered, ensuring that you and your patient are adequately informed about the reasoning behind these tests, as well as their practicalities.

This is followed by **organ-specific chapters**; the ear, nose, and throat are discussed individually, with each chapter laid out in the following order:

- Basic **anatomy:** the major anatomical structures and functional mechanisms which are key to the functioning of each organ.
- **Differential diagnoses:** this key page shows a symptom map with the symptoms a patient may present with.
- Each **condition** is then explored by **section**, from background through causes and investigations to management. This should make it easy to approach common yet potentially complex symptoms in the consultation room.

Pediatric ENT is covered in a similar manner, although the chapter is not split by organ.

And with that, you are ready to manage all common ear, nose, and throat presentations!

Chapter 1
Clinical assessment

1.1	How to take a focused history of the ear, nose, and throat	2
1.2	How to perform a clinical examination of the ear, nose, and throat	4
1.3	Investigations in ENT	7
1.4	ENT tests performed during the clinical examination	8
1.5	Specialist tests	10
1.6	Vestibular function tests	15
1.7	Other investigations used in ENT	17

1.1 How to take a focused history of the ear, nose, and throat

This chapter focuses on aspects of the history pertinent to the ENT system; however, this does not detract from the need to take a comprehensive history (see below for the basic layout of a presenting concern and history of the presenting illness).

| Presenting complaint and its history | Review of systems | Past medical and past surgical history | Allergies and medications history | Family history | Social history |

Each positive symptom will need to be explored and the presence of associated symptoms reviewed. It is important to remember to explore the patient's concerns and expectations.

1.1.1 Ear history

The following *symptoms* can occur in ear pathology (be sure to check if bilaterally):
- Ear pain, itching or irritation in the ear, discharge from the ear (if present, ask its color and screen for systemic symptoms), tinnitus, hearing loss, wax, dizziness / vertigo / off-balance sensation, facial asymmetry, difficulty articulating.

Be sure that you screen for the following *risk factors*:
- History of: trauma, noise exposure, flying
- Drug history, especially use of antibiotics or diuretics.

Of particular importance in the patient's *past history* and *social history*:
- Previous ENT surgery
- Medical co-morbidities including a history of atopy or allergy*
- Occupation and previous occupation, if any
- History of cigarette and alcohol use.

1.1.2 Nose history

The following *symptoms* can occur in nose pathology and it is important to explore the impact of these symptoms on speech and sleep:
- Nasal blockage, irritation in the nose, anterior nasal discharge (if present, ask its color), post-nasal discharge, epistaxis, facial pain or pressure, sneezing, snoring, sleep apnea; check for impairment in sense of smell or taste.

Be sure that you screen for the following *risk factors*:
- History of acute nasal or sinus infection (including any treatment used)
- Trauma.

Of particular importance in the patient's *past history* and *social history*:
- Previous ENT surgery
- Medical co-morbidities including a history of atopy or allergy*
- History of cigarette and alcohol use.

1.1.3 Throat history

The following *symptoms* can occur in throat pathology:
- Sensation of a foreign body in the throat, need to keep clearing the throat, weight loss, dysphagia, odynophagia (pain on swallowing), change in the voice, stridor, difficulty breathing, coughing, neck lumps.

Be sure that you screen for the following *risk factors*:
- History of: acid reflux / heartburn, previous tonsillitis / pharyngitis / laryngitis
- Dietary history and current eating habits
- Previous medication use.

Of particular importance in the patient's *past history* and *social history*:
- Previous surgery in the neck area, e.g. tonsillectomy / adenoidectomy / thyroidectomy
- Medical co-morbidities including a history of atopy or allergy*
- Occupation and previous occupation, if any
- History of cigarette and alcohol use.

---

*The majority of allergic patients have multiple allergies; when taking an allergy history be sure to ask about seasonal, perennial and occupational allergen exposure as well as food (especially nuts), drug and insect bite allergies. It is also very important to document prior drug use and immunization history to assist the management plan.

1.2 How to perform a clinical examination of the ear, nose, and throat

1.2.1 Ear examination

Equipment: gloves, otoscope, ear swab (if discharge present).

Inspection: begin by inspecting the pinna, surrounding skin (for rashes or erythema) and external auditory meatus.

Palpation: press on the mastoid process, which is located posteriorly and inferiorly to the ear. If this is tender it may indicate mastoiditis (see *Section 2.7.5*).

Otoscopy: hold the otoscope in the same hand as the ear you are examining, e.g. hold the otoscope in your left hand if you are examining the patient's left ear – see *Figure 1.1*.

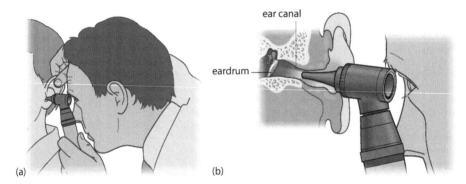

ear canal

eardrum

(a)   (b)

Figure 1.1 (a) The correct way to hold and insert an otoscope; (b) otoscope inserted into the ear canal as part of the examination.

Begin by checking for wax, debris or discharge in the canal. Then move on to the tympanic membrane: check its color and contour (from bulging to retracted), inspect all four quadrants of the membrane and check for the light reflex. Be sure you inspect for perforation of, or a fluid level behind, the tympanic membrane.

If you note any ear discharge present, use an ear swab to take a sample and send it to the laboratory for C&S (culture and sensitivity) or check for its glucose level (if clear and you suspect it to be cerebrospinal fluid (CSF), see *Section 2.12*).

1.2.2 Nose examination

Equipment: gloves, penlight (headlight in specialist clinic), nasal speculum or nasendoscope (in specialist clinics), specimen container (if available).

Inspection: look for any scars, deformities, deviation, swelling, or bruising of the nose.

Examination of the nostrils: when in non-specialist clinics use a penlight and the nasal speculum to examine each nostril – this is called anterior rhinoscopy. Hold the speculum in your left hand; it is balanced on the index finger with the middle and ring finger on either side of the speculum (used to modify the width of the speculum to allow for easy entry into the nostril) – see *Figure 1.2*.

If you do not have this speculum, the alternative is to ask the patient to tilt their head back, while you gently push the tip of the nose upward using your thumb and use an otoscope to examine each nostril.

Inspect for color of the nasal lining (e.g. blue if hyperemic), abnormalities of the nasal septum (e.g. deflection or a spur), bleeding or clotted blood (check for congestion around Little's area (also known as Kiesselbach's plexus) if history of epistaxis), discharge, any growths (e.g. polyps, whether unilateral or bilateral) or abnormality of the inferior turbinate (e.g. hypertrophy or cobblestone appearance).

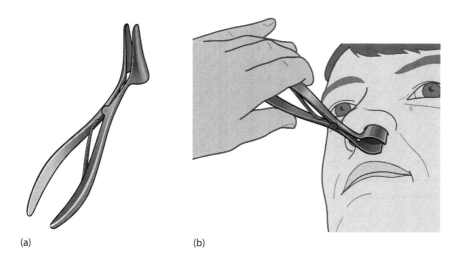

(a) (b)

Figure 1.2 (a) A nasal speculum; (b) speculum inserted into the nostril as part of the examination.

In specialist clinics, anterior rhinoscopy or flexible nasal endoscopy can be used; these provide a much greater view of the inside of the nose. As well as identifying the above pathology, the following can also be identified: abnormalities of the middle and superior turbinate (e.g. enlargement), Grade 1 nasal polyps (see below), any mass in the post-nasal space, the health of the Eustachian tube cushion, as well as indications the patient has had previous surgery on the nose or sinus. In addition, antrostomy can be seen under the inferior turbinate (indicative of previous sinus-related surgery) and anterior or middle ethmoid open cells (in those who have had previous nasal surgery).

Nasal polyps are inflammatory fluid-filled sacs, pale white in color; they can be seen during anterior rhinoscopy or nasal endoscopy. To differentiate between a nasal polyp and the inferior turbinate, a polyp can be fully circulated by the probe. If it is not a polyp (but is instead an enlarged inferior turbinate) the probe will not be able to pass on the lateral side (due to attachment of inferior turbinate to the lateral wall of the nose). Also, a nasal polyp is insensitive, meaning that on contact with the probe the patient will not feel pain. Touching the inferior turbinate, however, can be painful for the patient.

Nasal polyps are graded by the following system:
- Grade 1 is when a small amount of polypoid tissue is seen and it is confined to the middle meatus
- Grade 2 is where multiple polyps are seen within this area
- Grade 3 indicates nasal polyps that have spread beyond the middle meatus
- Grade 4 is when the nasal cavity is entirely blocked by nasal polyps.

1.2.3 Throat examination

Equipment: gloves, penlight (headlight in specialist clinic), tongue depressor, glass of water.

Inspection: inspect the neck for any swelling, look at the lips and surrounding skin, inside the mouth, dentition and tongue.

Palpation: if you detect a neck lump, identify its site, size, shape, color, any tenderness, its edges and consistency and any distinctive features, its mobility, and whether it is attached to the overlying skin. Determine its relationship to swallowing by asking the patient to take a sip of water and look, then feel, the lump as the patient swallows this sip. This will differentiate whether or not the lump arises in/is related to the thyroid.

Assess for any lymphadenopathy in the submental, submandibular, cervical, and pre- and post-auricular chains. Move to the oral cavity to examine dentition, tongue and gums. Use the tongue depressor to examine the tonsils and palate (palatal movement is assessed by asking the patient to say 'aaahhh').

NB: If you suspect the problem emanates from the thyroid gland (midline, associated goiter, moves on swallowing) then it is important to also carry out a systemic thyroid examination.

1.3 Investigations in ENT

Investigations are carried out based on the patient's symptoms and history. They are used to support the working diagnosis, exclude a potentially serious cause, and/or aid the initiation of definitive management.

1.3.1 Specialist hearing and speech tests: an overview

These are used to identify the affected ear, the hearing deficit at the time, the type of hearing loss, the pressure of the middle ear, and any speech impairment due to hearing loss.

Hearing tests can be subjective (relying on the patient's considered response) or objective (where the patient does not make a conscious decision, but instead their response is detected automatically using specialist equipment). The latter are done by specially-trained audiologists.

There are specialist laboratory tests which are used to assess the functioning of a patient's balance apparatus and brain function.

Radiological investigations, such as computerized tomography (CT) and magnetic resonance imaging (MRI) scans, are used to visualize structures within the petrous temporal bone.

1.4 ENT tests performed during the clinical examination

1.4.1 Speech test

This is a simple test and should be performed at primary care level as a screening test. It will identify whether the patient can discriminate between different sounds and will also test the patient's ability to recognize spoken words. The results of this test, in the context of the remainder of the assessment, will guide your management.

Procedure summary: the clinician will be required to state a phonetically balanced set of words, e.g. cup, cat, cart, tree, key, he, shop, shave, shelf, etc. whilst they have either a book or their hand in front of their mouth to prevent any lip reading by the patient. The patient should be able to repeat the words the clinician said to them.

1.4.2 Weber and Rinne tuning fork tests

This is another important test which can be performed at primary care level to differentiate between conductive and sensorineural hearing loss and to identify the affected ear.

Procedure summary for Weber test: hold the tuning fork in the dominant hand and strike it against a hard object (commonly against the clinician's flexed forearm, just distal to the elbow). The vibrating fork is then placed in the midline of the patient's head. Ask the patient if they hear the sound left, right or center?

- Hearing the sound in the midline or center is a normal response.
- Hearing the sound louder in the good ear, indicates a sensorineural hearing loss (SNHL) in the affected ear.
- Hearing the sound louder in the ear with the hearing loss indicates a conductive hearing loss (CHL) in the affected ear.

Procedure summary for Rinne test: the clinician may activate the tuning fork again as needed. The tuning fork is then held on the mastoid bone to check for bone conduction (BC). Ask the patient if they hear the tuning fork. If the patient does, then hold the tuning fork just lateral to the opening of the external ear canal to check for air conduction (AC). Ask the patient if it is louder:

- If the sound is louder at the EAC opening of the affected ear, a SNHL is indicated.
- If the sound is louder on the mastoid of the affected ear, a CHL is indicated.

If the test is performed on someone with normal hearing bilaterally, the patient will hear the sound midline on the Weber test and air conduction is heard better than bone conduction.

The tests are documented as follows (see *Table 1.1*):

- Weber: midline, or lateralizes to left or right.
- Rinne: AC > BC, or BC > AC.

The tests may be performed post-operatively to evaluate hearing loss.

Post-operatively, doctors rely on the Weber test to assess the success of the operation and exclude a deaf ear.

Table 1.1 Interpretation of Weber and Rinne tests

Rinne test right ear	Rinne test left ear	Weber test	Diagnosis
AC > BC	AC > BC	Midline	Normal hearing bilaterally (could also signify a bilaterally symmetrical SNHL)
BC > AC	AC > BC	Right	Conductive hearing loss, right ear
AC > BC	BC > AC	Left	Conductive hearing loss, left ear
AC > BC	AC > BC	Right	Sensorineural hearing loss left ear
AC > BC	AC > BC	Left	Sensorineural hearing loss right ear

AC = air conduction; BC = bone conduction.

1.5 Specialist tests

1.5.1 Pure tone audiogram

The pure tone audiogram is a key audiological test for assessing hearing and is carried out by specialist audiologists. Primary care clinicians may recommend audiology evaluation or refer to Otolaryngology (ENT) for hearing evaluation.

This test is a psychoacoustic test which determines the subject's pure tone threshold. By producing pure tones that can be varied by frequency and intensity, the audiogram produced is a plot of frequency against intensity, measured in decibels (dB). Both the nerve and bone conduction thresholds are measured to ascertain the nature of the deficit.

Procedure summary: this test is performed in a soundproof room by an audiologist or, occasionally, by a trained hearing specialist. In this room, the patient is asked to wear headphones which are plugged into an audiometer. The audiologist is sitting on the other side and they control the machine which will, upon their direction, produce a clicking sound at varying frequencies. If the patient hears the sound they respond by pressing on a buzzer. These responses will then be mapped to produce an audiogram, the graphic result of the responses. This represents air conduction.

To test bone conduction (the sensorineural part of hearing) instead, a small vibrator (attached to the same audiometer) is pressed against the patient's mastoid process. The vibrations from the device transmit directly to the inner ear, bypassing the ear canal and middle ear. The patient's responses are recorded as sensorineural responses and mapped as above.

Interpretation: this test measures how loud sound has to be for a person to hear, this being representative of the functioning of the auditory pathway. The audiogram is used to determine the type, degree, and configuration of the hearing loss. *Figure 1.3* is an example of what the results from an audiogram look like; note that audiologists administering the test will often interpret the results and present their assessment in their report.

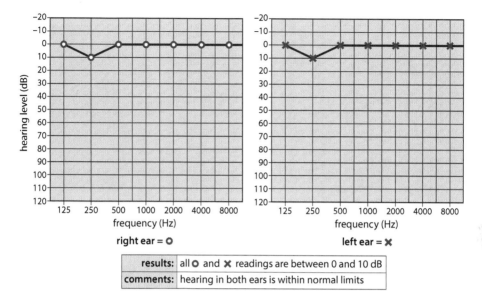

right ear = O

left ear = ✖

results:	all O and ✖ readings are between 0 and 10 dB
comments:	hearing in both ears is within normal limits

Figure 1.3 Audiogram results showing normal hearing in both ears.

The amount of hearing loss, in decibels, can be equated to a Grade of hearing loss. This has implications on the impact the hearing loss may be having on day-to-day activity, detailed in *Table 1.2*. Test results of 0–10 dB are regarded as excellent hearing and up to 25 dB is regarded as being around the threshold for normal hearing. After this is hearing loss territory: 25–45 dB is regarded as mild hearing loss which will have some effects on day-to-day hearing; 45–65 dB is regarded as moderate hearing loss impacting day-to-day conversation; 65–85 dB is seen as severe hearing loss, and a loss of greater than 85 dB is profound hearing loss.

Table 1.2 Severity of hearing loss with associated impairment

Hearing level (dB)	Result
0–10	Excellent hearing
10–25	Normal hearing above threshold level
25–45	Mild hearing loss *Missing some aspects of conversation but managing well*
45–65	Moderate hearing loss *Patient may be missing out in day-to-day conversation; consider intervention*
65–85	Severe hearing loss *Not able to manage any conversation*
>85	Profound hearing loss

1.5.2 Tympanogram

This test is carried out by specialists – it measures the external ear canal volume and best compliance of the tympanic membrane by equating it with the middle ear pressure.

Procedure summary: in this technique, an airtight soft-tipped probe, containing a small microphone and a fine tube connected to an air pressure pump, is inserted into the ear canal. It is an objective, non-invasive, and quick test (typically only lasting a few minutes).

Interpretation: the sound-conducting properties of the middle ear are measured and the readings produce a graph with a bell-shaped curve, where the peak of the curve is close to the normal atmospheric pressure. The data and graph will be interpreted by the specialist conducting the exam and their interpretation will be stated in the report.

In short, type A (*Figure 1.4*) implies normal middle ear pressure. Type B, seen as a flat curve, is due to splinting of the tympanic membrane, usually by fluid in the middle ear. Type C implies negative middle ear pressure due to dysfunction of the Eustachian tube. Other abnormalities include cases where the ossicles of the middle ear are not connected to each other (ossicular discontinuity), due to trauma or chronic infection, when the peak of the graph can be very high. Conversely, if the ossicles are fused together such as in otosclerosis, the peak of the graph is often reduced in height, although still in the normal pressure range.

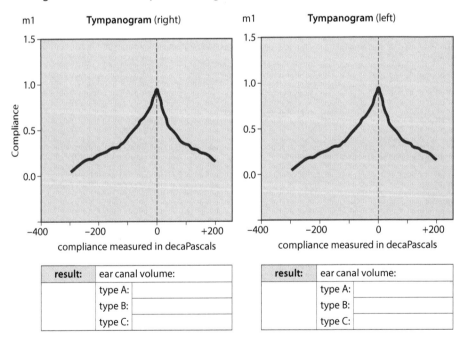

Figure 1.4 Tympanogram showing normal results.

1.5.3 Speech audiogram

This is a highly skilled test requested by ENT specialists in conjunction with the audiogram. It is carried out by specially trained audiologists in a specialized audiology clinic.

The basis of this test is word recognition by the patient, tolerance of speech stimuli, degree and type of hearing loss. It measures the actual disability produced by the hearing and it examines the discrimination ability above threshold.

One of its routine uses is in the pre-operative assessment for stapedectomy in otosclerosis, where it is important to know the level of the gain in hearing from such surgery. This test can also be used by specialists to support or be used as a specialized investigation to reach the diagnosis. Speech audiograms are used diagnostically in the US to evaluate for discrepancies in speech discrimination.

Procedure summary: extensive knowledge on the formal procedure goes beyond the scope of this section. However, in the 'live speech' version of this test the patient is asked to sit in a soundproof room, with the examiner in an adjacent room, and an audiometer with microphones in both rooms is used by the audiologists to carry out this test.

Interpretation: this is a specialty test, performed and evaluated by audiologists or otolaryngology specialists. The results in the context of the full assessment will be released back to the referring team and primary care.

Note that if the findings of the speech audiometry are not consistent with the pure tone audiogram, further investigation is warranted, in order to see if there is an element of auditory processing disorder, or even malingering. This would require further investigations including otoacoustic emissions (see *Section 1.5.5*), acoustic reflexes and auditory brainstem-evoked response (see *Section 1.5.4*) which would exclude more subtle peripheral disease.

1.5.4 Auditory brainstem-evoked response

The auditory brainstem response (ABR) or brainstem auditory evoked response (BAER) is a specialist test, and is the most objective test to detect hearing loss. It has high specificity and sensitivity and is used to detect hearing loss in children as young as three months old. In the US it is sometimes performed in newborns to evaluate for possible congenital hearing loss. Typically, otoacoustic emission tests are performed on each newborn in a hospital, with further evaluation with ABR/BAER as indicated. This test assesses the inner ear pathway (see *Section 2.1*); as the cochlea detects sound waves it converts these into electrical signals which are transmitted to the auditory area in the brain via the eighth cranial nerve.

Procedure summary: electrodes are placed on different points on the head of the patient which will detect the electrical potentials being generated from the inner ear heading towards the auditory area of the brain. As the electrodes detect these, the data is entered into a specialized computer system.

Interpretation: this is a specialized test and as such, interpretation is limited to the trained audiologists who work with the data and system to produce a report of the results.

1.5.5 Otoacoustic emission

This is one of the most objective and sensitive tests for hearing. It is based on the principle that in the normal inner ear the cochlea will produce specific emissions as it is stimulated to generate sound by movement of the hair cells. These emissions can be detected through the procedure described below. Patients with hearing loss (>25 dB) do not produce these soft emissions.

Additionally, this test can detect blockage of the outer ear canal, the middle ear pressure, and whether there is damage to the hair cells in the cochlea. It can be used in newborns to detect their hearing.

Procedure summary: the audiologist and patient are sitting in the same room, and a soft probe is inserted into the ear canal with its wire leading to a computer. The data received from the probe is analyzed by the software system.

Interpretation: this is a specialized test and as such, interpretation is limited to the trained audiologists who work with the data and system to produce a report of the results.

1.6 Vestibular function tests

Pure dizziness is usually investigated in specialist clinics in secondary care. However, primary care plays an important role in ensuring that the presenting concern is not syncope or presyncope which would require investigations along the lines of blood tests, electrocardiogram (ECG) and/or echocardiogram.

1.6.1 Caloric test

This is a specialist test and is a very important investigation utilizing the nystagmus seen clinically in response to stimuli. Nystagmus is a sudden jerky movement of the eyes and has two components: slow and fast. The test measures vestibular function and provides information about loss of function of a unilateral semicircular canal or directional preponderance (non-specific enhancement of nystagmus in one direction suggests a usually non-localizing pathology).

Procedure summary: each ear is stimulated alternately with air at 30°C and then 44°C for 40 seconds, and the duration of nystagmus is measured from onset of nystagmus to fading, by recording time (the test can also be performed by irrigating with warm and cool water, but this produces more nausea than air stimulation and is rarely performed at this time). The direction of nystagmus is described by its fast component.

Interpretation: in those with Ménière's disease or an acoustic neuroma, there is reduced or absent reaction to cold and warm water stimuli in the ipsilateral eye to the affected ear. A prolonged response indicates an irritable labyrinth.

1.6.2 Electronystagmography

Electronystagmography (ENG, or videonystagmography (VNG)) is a specialist care test used to assess various aspects of the balance system. It is done in conjunction with the caloric test, especially for those with concurrent balance symptoms.

Procedure summary: some preparation is required in advance; patients may be asked to withhold the medication they take for vertigo or sedatives for the preceding 3–5 days. Patients are advised not to wear excessive facial makeup on the day of the test, to ensure good electrode contact with the skin.

This test is carried out in a darkened room where the patient watches a moving light. As the eyes move away from the line of straight gaze these movements are noted and recorded automatically by sensors placed on the side of the eyes and forehead, or by using special goggles. The changes in electrical potential are used to follow the pattern of nystagmus reactions.

Interpretation: the data from the test is analyzed by specialist computer programs and those trained to administer the test and will be reported back as either normal or abnormal. In the context of the remainder of the assessment it is used by specialist teams to identify the cause of the dizziness and further management.

1.6.3 Computerized dynamic posturography testing (Equi test)

Posturography, a highly specialized test, is an objective measurement of how the patient can cope with day-to-day activities in the context of their balance disturbance.

Procedure summary: in this test, the patient is required to stand on a platform for approximately 15 minutes. During the test, the platform or surrounding screen may move.

Interpretation: the results from the test are interpreted by specialist services who commission the test. One example of its use is in vestibular rehabilitation programs where it is done before and after rehabilitation to assess the impact of the therapy.

1.7 Other investigations used in ENT

Ear swabs are used if there is ear discharge present.

- The swab can be sent for microbe culture and sensitivity to identify causative pathogens and which antibiotics they are sensitive to.
- If there is clear discharge, then it can be tested for glucose to exclude CSF leak.

Syphilis serology can be requested if risk factors are found in the initial assessment. Secondary and tertiary syphilis may both cause sudden or chronic hearing loss in one or both ears, in addition to impairment in balance. The most sensitive evaluation for tertiary syphilis is the fluorescent treponemal antibody (FTA) absorption test.

1.7.1 Radiology

Imaging commonly requested, when investigating for acoustic neuroma, cerebellopontine angle lesion, and cholesteatoma, is typically a gadolinium-enhanced magnetic resonance imaging (MRI) scan of the internal auditory canal (IAC) and brain. If there are contraindications to having an MRI scan (e.g. pacemaker, cochlear implant, some joint replacements or metal inside the body) then a computerized tomography (CT) scan can be performed; however, the resultant information may be comparatively limited.

Neck lumps should be investigated based upon the working diagnosis; see *Section 4.15*.

1.7.2 Ultrasound scan of the neck +/– fine needle aspiration

Procedure summary: an ultrasound machine (which has monitors on top of the central machine, with the ultrasound probe attached to this via a wire) uses sound waves to identify characteristics of the body part being imaged. A transparent gel is applied to the area of neck in question and the ultrasound probe is moved along this, with the radiologist reviewing the images. It is usually a painless procedure. There is no preparation required for this test. Ultrasound is frequently used to evaluate the thyroid gland if indicated.

At times, the ultrasound scan can be used as a guide to help the interventional radiologist to take samples from the neck lump, using the technique of fine needle aspiration (FNA). Local anesthetic is injected just under the skin overlying the neck lump and then the ultrasound scan machine and probe are used as above. When the interventional radiologist feels they have an appropriate site, a thin needle is inserted and a sample of the lump is withdrawn; this can then be sent to the lab for cytology or histopathology.

Interpretation: the radiologist (reviewing the ultrasound images) and histopathologist (reviewing the cytology) will provide a report to the doctor requesting the investigation.

1.7.3 Sialogram

Procedure summary: this is an X-ray-based procedure to assess the salivary glands and tract. The patient will lie on a bed in the X-ray room in the radiology department, and a small tube will be inserted into the opening of the salivary gland duct (located at the floor of the mouth for the submandibular gland and in the cheek for the parotid). Patients may find this uncomfortable but it shouldn't be painful.

Contrast (a colorless liquid) is then introduced to the tube and X-rays are taken (X-rays may also be taken before the contrast is introduced, unless there are some already available on the system). The contrast is not dangerous to ingest but all possible measures are taken to avoid this. The tube will then be removed and the patient will be asked to ingest a bitter solution to help drain the contrast from the glands; some X-rays may also be taken at this time.

There is no specific preparation needed by the patient prior to the examination; however, it should be noted that before the procedure the patient may be asked to remove earrings, necklaces, dentures and even hearing aids.

Interpretation: the report from the radiologists will be sent to the referring doctor.

Chapter 2
Ear

2.1	Basic anatomy of the ear	20
2.2	Differential diagnosis of ear problems	23
2.3	Deafness and hearing loss	25
2.4	Sudden hearing loss	28
2.5	Wax	30
2.6	Otitis externa	31
2.7	Otitis media	33
2.8	Cholesteatoma	36
2.9	Perforation of the tympanic membrane	38
2.10	Otosclerosis	40
2.11	Acoustic neuroma	43
2.12	The draining ear	45
2.13	Earache	47
2.14	Vertigo and dizziness	49
2.15	Benign paroxysmal positional vertigo	51
2.16	Labyrinthitis	53
2.17	Ménière's disease	55
2.18	Tinnitus	58
2.19	Presbycusis	60
2.20	Facial paralysis	61
2.21	Foreign body in the ear	65
2.22	Furuncle in the external auditory canal	66

2.1 Basic anatomy of the ear

The ear consists of three parts (external, middle and inner), as shown in *Figure 2.1*.

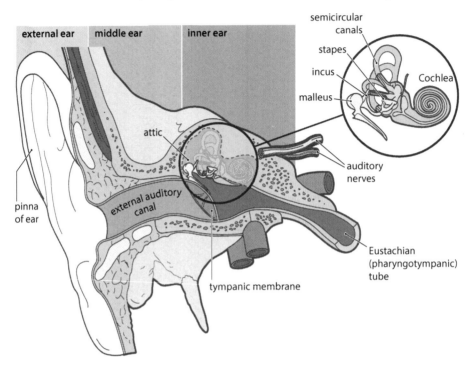

Figure 2.1 Ear anatomy.
Reproduced from *Anatomy and Physiology in Healthcare*, © Scion Publishing Ltd, 2017.

2.1.1 External ear

The external ear begins with the pinna which funnels sound waves from the environment to the external auditory meatus (canal). The external auditory canal (EAC) is approximately 3.2 cm in length and 0.6 cm in diameter. This canal has an outer cartilaginous part and an inner bony part (part of the temporal bone). The canal is slightly curved, with its outer part (outer one-third) containing hair follicles and ceruminous glands (which produce wax), both working to protect against infection, insects, trauma and foreign bodies. Importantly, the canal maintains the necessary temperature and humidity required to ensure elasticity of the tympanic membrane.

2.1.2 Middle ear

The tympanic membrane is where the external ear ends medially; in the healthy state the tympanic membrane appears gray–pink in color and is supported in the tympanic ring by the malleus (one of the three ossicle bones found in the middle ear). The tympanic membrane is made up of three layers: the outermost (or lateral) layer of tympanic membrane is modified skin of the external auditory canal, the middle layer is made of the radical and circular fibers, and the internal (or innermost) layer is formed of a mucous membrane which is continuous with the middle ear mucous membrane.

When a sound wave hits the tympanic membrane it causes it to vibrate and this vibration is transmitted to the ossicles (the name given to three small bones present in the middle ear, called the malleus, incus and stapes (see the insert in *Figure 2.1*), but often referred to as the hammer, anvil and footplate, respectively). The ossicles transmit vibrations from the tympanic membrane to the cochlea in the inner ear. This is because the base of the stapes bone (the most medial of the three bones) fits into the oval window (part of the cochlea). The cochlea converts those vibrations to sound signals (in the form of electrical energy) which are transmitted along the cranial nerve to the brain, producing the sense of hearing. The round window is one of the two openings in the medial wall of the middle ear; it leads to the cochlea and is covered by a secondary tympanic membrane.

Although only 2 cm³ in volume, the middle ear cavity, lined with mucous membrane, has several key relations: the lateral wall of this cavity is formed by the tympanic membrane, the medial wall contains the bulge of the facial nerve and the floor is separated from the internal jugular vein by only a thin plate of bone. Its roof separates the middle ear from the middle cranial fossa. Posteriorly is the aditus (the opening to mastoid air cells), and anteriorly is the Eustachian tube, which is a connection between the middle ear and the lateral wall of the posterior nasal space.

The function of the Eustachian tube is to maintain middle ear pressure and ventilate the cavity. Normally this tube is closed but it opens with each swallow to carry out its function of equalizing pressure in the middle ear cavity. There are two muscles in the middle ear cavity: the stapedius and the tensor tympani, which protect the inner ear from loud noise trauma by contracting on exposure to loud noise.

2.1.3 Inner ear

The inner ear contains the cochlea and vestibular system, both of which are contained in the same bony capsule and share the same liquids: endolymph and perilymph. This fluid moves as we move our head to different positions, and the movement of the fluid is sensed by tiny hairs in the semicircular canals which send messages to the brain, thereby helping to maintain balance and posture.

The cochlea is the so-called 'hearing organ' and is shaped like a snail (see *Figure 2.2*). It consists of three liquid-filled tubes; the innermost tube is called the cochlear duct and it secretes endolymph. The cochlear duct contains the basilar membrane, on which lies the organ of Corti, a sensory organ containing hair cells attached to sensory nerves which are responsible for hearing. The most curled part of the cochlea (the innermost part) is responsible for the lower frequency sounds, while the basal end (the proximal or outermost part) is responsible for higher frequency impulses. The auditory branch of the eighth cranial nerve carries impulses to the brainstem and temporal lobe in the cerebral cortex.

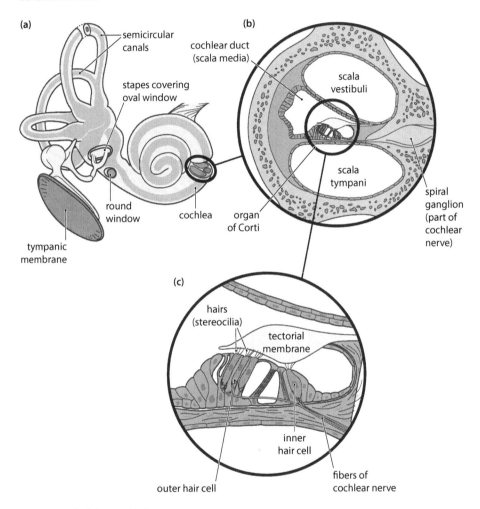

Figure 2.2 Cochlear and balance apparatus.
Reproduced from *Anatomy and Physiology in Healthcare*, © Scion Publishing Ltd, 2017.

The balance apparatus comprises the three semicircular canals found in each ear; these are responsible for maintaining balance in relation to gravity and position of the head. They respond to rotational movement. These canals are supplied by the eighth cranial nerve – vestibular branch. The canals open into the vestibule, which is an oval chamber and contains the utricle and saccule (these are otolith organs) which function to sense motion. The utricle detects movement in the horizontal plane (linear acceleration, either forward–backward or left–right), while the saccule detects movement in the vertical plane, i.e. up–down.

2.2 Differential diagnosis of ear problems

After performing a clinical assessment of the patient, consisting of the history and physical examination shown in *Sections 1.1* and *1.2*, a differential diagnosis based on the symptoms shown in the left-hand column can be considered. The presenting symptoms are shown in order of prevalence in terms of causative pathology for the index symptom.

Symptom	Differential diagnosis	Section number
Ear drainage	Eczema, psoriasis or dermatitis of the external auditory canal	*Section 2.12*
	Otitis externa	*Section 2.6*
	Boil in the ear	*Section 2.22*
	Mastoiditis	*Section 2.7.5*
	OM +/– cholesteatoma formation	*Section 2.7*
	Perforation of the tympanic membrane	*Section 2.9*
	Trauma	*Section 2.12*
	Foreign body in the ear	*Section 2.21*
Ear pain	Boil in the ear	*Section 2.22*
	OM (serous and acute)	*Section 2.7*
	Otitis externa (acute)	*Section 2.6*
	Mastoiditis	*Section 2.7.5*
	Wax/cerumen	*Section 2.5*
	Foreign body in the ear	*Section 2.21*
	Ramsay Hunt syndrome	*Section 2.20*
	Referred ear pain	*Section 2.13*
Hearing loss	Wax/cerumen	*Section 2.5*
	OM (serous, acute, and chronic suppurative)	*Section 2.7*
	Foreign body in the ear	*Section 2.21*
	Mastoiditis	*Section 2.7.5*
	Perforation of the tympanic membrane	*Section 2.9*
	Otitis externa	*Section 2.6*
	Otosclerosis	*Section 2.10*
	Presbycusis	*Section 2.19*
	Ménière's disease	*Section 2.17*
	Acoustic neuroma	*Section 2.11*
	Please see Section 2.3 *for all other causes*	
	Please see Section 2.4 *for Sudden hearing loss*	

Symptom	Differential diagnosis	Section number
Tinnitus	Loud noise exposure	*Section 2.18*
	Acute perforation of tympanic membrane	*Section 2.9*
	OM (serous)	*Section 2.7*
	Eustachian tube dysfunction	*Section 2.18*
	Viral upper respiratory tract infection	*Section 2.18*
	Hearing loss	*Section 2.3*
	Anxiety / stress	*Section 2.18*
	Trauma to the head	*Section 2.18*
	Otosclerosis	*Section 2.10*
	Wax/cerumen	*Section 2.5*
	Foreign body in the ear	*Section 2.21*
	Acoustic neuroma	*Section 2.11*
	Ramsay Hunt syndrome	*Section 2.20*
	Please see Section 2.4 for Sudden hearing loss	
Vertigo (acoustic neuroma)	Benign positional paroxysmal vertigo	*Section 2.15*
	Labyrinthitis and vestibular neuronitis	*Section 2.16*
	Ménière's disease	*Section 2.17*
	Migraine	*Section 2.14*
Facial paralysis* (acoustic neuroma affecting CN VII)	Ramsay Hunt syndrome	*Section 2.20*
	Bell's palsy	*Section 2.20*
	Cholesteatoma	*Section 2.8*
	Malignant growth	*Section 2.20*

*Although this is not an ear symptom in itself, the diseases which may cause this and have consequences on the ear, are listed here.

2.3 Deafness and hearing loss

Deafness is the inability to hear and understand sounds. It can affect people of any age group and can be either unilateral or bilateral in nature. The anatomical location of the lesion causes either a conductive or sensorineural hearing loss, although patients could have either one or mixed pictures.

In **conductive hearing loss**, there is a defect in the conduction of sound along the pathway to the cochlea. The lesion causing conductive hearing loss may be anywhere: the external auditory meatus, external auditory canal, tympanic membrane, Eustachian tube, ossicular chain in the middle ear cavity, and/or footplate of stapes at the oval window (see *Section 2.1*).

Any pathology beyond the oval window causing deafness is termed **sensorineural hearing loss**. This can include dysfunction of the cochlear and/or the auditory nerve which supplies the hair cells in the organ of Corti and the sensory fibers of which lead to the brainstem.

2.3.1 Clinical assessment

A focused history (see *Section 1.1*), clinical examination including otoscopy (see *Section 1.2*) and tuning fork test (see *Section 1.4.2*) will be helpful in guiding you toward the likely diagnosis and initial management.

2.3.2 Causes of conductive hearing loss and findings on examination

Some of the most common causes are described below together with their findings on examination; these can be elicited clinically – see above.

Wax/cerumen impaction	Wax/cerumen appears golden brown or amber in color when it is soft, and dark brown or even black when hard.
Foreign body	In adults, most common are pieces of cotton-tipped applicators, commonly known as 'Q-tips'. In children, building block pieces, beads, popcorn or insects.
OM (acute)	A red congested tympanic membrane with a fluid level or air bubble behind the tympanic membrane.
OM (serous)	A fluid level or fluid 'bubbles' are seen behind the tympanic membrane, though not as red as when acute.
Eustachian tube dysfunction	A retracted eardrum is seen, with or without a fluid level. The tympanic membrane may appear normal.

Mastoiditis	Tenderness on palpation of the mastoid region behind the ear, and there may also be erythema and edema of the mastoid area. A congested tympanic membrane is seen on otoscopy.
Barotrauma	This will be seen as a retracted eardrum with a distorted shape.
Keratosis obturans	This is a collection of desquamated (shed) skin visualized in the external auditory canal.
Exostosis of the external auditory canal	Bony growths generally found along the suture lines of the bones of the external auditory canal. They may accumulate excessive skin and keratinized tissue and, if large, cause conductive hearing loss.
Osteoma of the external auditory canal	A bony swelling in the medial half of the external auditory canal can be visualized.
Chronic suppurative OM +/− cholesteatoma	Pus-like discharge with squamous debris in the external and middle ear with attic defect.
Perforated tympanic membrane	A hole can be seen in the tympanic membrane. If this hole is in the center of the eardrum it is regarded as safe perforation, whereas if around the margin of the eardrum, especially at the attic, it is unsafe and should be checked for cholesteatoma under the microscope.
Malignant otitis externa	Discharge and debris seen in the external auditory canal, with or without exposed bone. This is a dangerous condition and must be distinguished from the more common otitis externa. Patients typically have a history of diabetes mellitus or are otherwise immunocompromised.
Otosclerosis	No specific findings are seen on examination of the ear.
Trauma to head leading to deafness	Hemotympanum (blood behind the tympanic membrane) seen as a purplish hue behind the tympanic membrane with fluid level.
Glomus tumor in the middle ear	A purplish glow is seen behind the tympanic membrane with no fluid level.

2.3.3 Causes of sensorineural hearing loss

There will be risk factors elicited in the history with minimal findings on examination.

Most common	Noise-induced
	Presbycusis
	Sudden onset sensorineural hearing loss (usually unknown etiology)
	Ototoxicity secondary to medications • e.g. aminoglycosides (causes destruction of cochlear hair cells, gentamicin being the most potent), furosemide, ethacrynic acid, salicylate (the ototoxic effect of large doses of salicylates is usually reversible) and chemotherapy
Least common	Trauma to the head • damage to the inner ear, temporal bone and/or base of skull
	Ménière's disease
	Acoustic neuroma
	Idiopathic

See *Section 2.2* for disease-specific management. All other causes not individually covered may require a referral to specialist ENT services.

2.3.4 Essential facts

Investigating for a cerebellopontine angle lesion

Arrange an audiogram (see *Section 1.5.1* for further details). With a sensorineural hearing loss >10 dB between the right and left ear in three consecutive frequencies a gadolinium-enhanced MRI of the internal auditory canal is indicated to rule out cerebellopontine angle lesions such as an acoustic neuroma.

Traumatic rupture of the round window after strenuous exercise, heavy weight lifting or sudden pressure changes (referred to as an inner ear fistula) can present with tinnitus, hearing loss and unsteadiness. Diagnosis can only be confirmed on tympanotomy. Plugging the hole with fat is the treatment of choice. There is no significant improvement with antivertiginous or vasodilator drugs.

Abnormal bony growth

Exostosis is hyperostosis of the tympanic bone (part of the external auditory canal) and is caused by a periosteal reaction to cold water, usually from swimming. **Osteomas** are uncommon benign tumors of the bone which usually arise from the tympanosquamous and tympanomastoid suture line.

Surgical treatment is recommended for both exostosis and osteoma in symptomatic patients (those with otalgia, conductive hearing loss or frequent ear infections).

2.4 Sudden hearing loss

2.4.1 Introduction

A sudden decrease in hearing is an **ENT emergency**. It usually affects one ear, being either conductive, sensorineural or mixed hearing loss picture. It may present with or without vertigo and/or tinnitus.

2.4.2 Diagnosis

The usual accepted definition of sudden hearing loss is hearing loss of more than 30 dB averaged over three frequencies and occurring within three days, although clinically it usually occurs over a period of minutes to hours. Also, consider this diagnosis in any patient who notes a subjective hearing loss of new onset and unexplained etiology.

There may be risk factors in the history which may indicate the etiology of the hearing loss; however, clinical examination is usually unremarkable.

2.4.3 Causes

Causes of hearing loss are listed below, from more to less common. It is noted that only 10–15% of people with sudden hearing loss have an identifiable cause.
- Wax or foreign body in the ear
- Serous OM
- Severe middle ear infection or cholesteatoma invading the inner ear
- Barotrauma / acoustic trauma / blast exposure
- Viral or bacterial labyrinthitis
- Ramsay Hunt syndrome
- Trauma involving temporal bone
- Stroke
- Acoustic neuroma
- Idiopathic
- Meningitis or mumps
- Ototoxicity
- Autoimmune disease of the inner ear.

2.4.4 Investigations

Tympanometry: see *Section 1.5.2* for further details. If tall peaked waves are shown, this is consistent with ossicular discontinuity. If the peak is flat, then this may indicate a middle ear effusion. A large volume on tympanometry (>2 ml) may indicate an invisible TM perforation.

Blood tests: these are to establish infective or systemic causes: complete blood count (CBC) with complete metabolic panel (CMP) covers kidney and liver function along with electrolytes, blood glucose level, thyroid function test (TFT), erythrocyte sedimentation rate (ESR), angiotensin-converting enzymes (ACE), antineutrophil cytoplasmic antibodies (ANCA), syphilis serology and viral titers (on first presentation and repeated after 6 weeks).

Specialist tests

These can be used to identify the cause, including **audiogram** (see *Section 1.5.1*), **speech audiogram** (see *Section 1.5.3*), **otoacoustic emission** (see *Section 1.5.5*), **auditory brainstem-evoked response** (see *Section 1.5.4*) – to evaluate inner ear function, and **MRI scan** of the head involving petrous temporal bone (see *Section 1.7.1*) – to exclude an acoustic neuroma; or CT if MRI contraindicated.

2.4.5 Management

Treatment should be targeted to the identified cause; it is important to determine if the hearing loss is conductive, sensorineural or mixed in nature. Treatments are controversial in the US because the benefits of interventions are unclear. However, treating with oral corticosteroids is generally recommended for patients with sensorineural hearing loss unless there are contraindications to systemic steroids. With failure to improve after 10 days of treatment, intratympanic steroids are recommended by experts. Antivirals were previously recommended, but have gone out of favor in the last several years. About 60% of patients receiving any form of active treatment improve on treatment; this is the same percentage as those who improve spontaneously. Current evidence indicates use of systemic steroids is not greater than spontaneous recovery rates.

2.4.6 Essential facts

All patients should be seen within 24 hours. When in primary care it is imperative that urgent ENT review is organized.

Patients with sudden onset sensorineural hearing loss should receive as soon as possible (ASAP) referral to otolaryngology for audiometry, evaluation, and treatment. Speech audiometry should be used to monitor any improvement or deterioration of the hearing, or its stability.

2.5 Wax

2.5.1 Introduction

Wax, also known as cerumen, is naturally produced in the external ear canal (see *Section 2.1*). The temporomandibular joint (TMJ) forms part of the anterior wall of the external auditory canal, and the movement of this joint helps to propel wax outward, toward the external auditory meatus.

If wax accumulates within the ear it can lead to a conductive hearing loss, earache, and tinnitus.

Some people are at increased risk of impaction of wax and the related consequences. This may be due to outflow obstruction of the wax (caused by, for example, using hearing aids, earplugs, or cotton buds) or patient-related factors such as a hairy or narrow ear canal.

2.5.2 Diagnosis

On otoscopy in the clinical examination (see *Section 1.2.1*), the offending wax can be seen. When soft it is golden in color; however, when hard or impacted it may appear dark brown or even black.

2.5.3 Management

Hydrogen peroxide or commercially available carbamide peroxide (Debrox) may be used by the patient at home with follow-up in primary care or otolaryngology. If there is a history of perforation of eardrum, previous ear surgery or PE tubes (also known as grommets) in the ear, then syringing or microsuction in the otolaryngology clinic may be carried out.

Patients who have a hairy external canal and suffer with excess production of wax should be advised to use olive oil once or twice a week routinely because wax can become entangled in the hairs where it dries, making it difficult for it to come out. This can ultimately impact on aeration of the ear canal and lead to infections such as otitis externa, and reduction in hearing.

When patients suffer from TMJ arthralgia (meaning they may stop chewing food on the affected side), this may lead to inadequate wax clearance on the affected side. These patients are more prone to blocked ears because of wax and otitis externa. Such patients need to make regular use of olive oil drops and follow-up in primary care or otolaryngology for suction when required.

2.6 Otitis externa

2.6.1 Introduction

Otitis externa is the umbrella term used to describe the many different causes of inflammation of the external auditory canal.

2.6.2 Diagnosis

The clinical history may reveal clues to the etiology with presenting concerns of pressure, pain, hearing loss, and/or drainage.

Examination will show debris in the external auditory meatus and tenderness, especially with traction on the pinna. Purulent yellow/greenish drainage indicates a bacterial infection whereas a creamy cheesy drainage on examination with black or white dust is indicative of fungal spores, and patients will require the appropriate treatment (see *Section 2.6.5*).

2.6.3 Causes

The most common causes are:
* Infections: bacterial (commonly *Staphylococcus*) or fungal (*Candida*, *Aspergillus*)
* Eczema or local allergic reaction to manufactured products, e.g. shampoos.

2.6.4 Investigations

Diagnosis can usually be made from clinical history and examination.

Tuning fork tests (see *Section 1.4.2*): may reveal a conductive hearing loss.

Ear swab: may obtain sample for C&S if there is ear drainage present, however, this is rarely done.

2.6.5 Management

Treatment takes the form of ear drops and/or rarely oral antibiotics.

Consider a **fungal infection** (see *Section 2.6.2*) in all cases of acute otitis externa that fail to resolve after appropriate treatment with topical antibiotics. Treatment is with topical antifungals such as clotrimazole, and the patient must be told the importance of water precautions for the ear. Consider early referral to otolaryngology because microsuction of the canal can be crucial in the treatment. Continue antifungal ear drops for one further week after improvement of their symptoms, which can take up to three weeks.

Otitis externa due to eczema of the external auditory canal is a difficult disease to cure, but symptomatic relief, reduction of severity of the symptoms, and attempts to delay or stop recurrence can be provided. In this condition patients commonly suffer from frequent watery ear discharge with severe itching. In the early stages, examination of the ear may show a normal external auditory canal. However, later it may appear dry and scaly, or in some cases moist and inflamed. If the ear becomes infected, then discharge and debris can be visualized, which needs microsuction in a hospital setting and a course of antibiotics and steroid-based ear drops. Syringing of the ear is not recommended in otitis externa as it can be extremely painful for the patient. Syringing will spread the infection and can cause perforation of the eardrum; mometasone ointment applied to the ear may be particularly effective as the petroleum base is lubricating and soothing.

Malignant otitis externa is one of the most severe forms of external ear canal infection. It is a form of osteomyelitis of the temporal bone. In this condition, the patient develops recurrent ear infection with debris and discharge. Consider the diagnosis of malignant otitis externa in any patient with diabetes or other immunocompromise and failure of appropriate treatment of otitis externa. Early referral to a specialist is appropriate because these patients often require inpatient care for intravenous antibiotics and suctioning of the ear canal. Concurrent management of the underlying condition (most commonly diabetes) is critical to successful treatment. Patients who are non-responsive to topical treatment may require a CT scan of petrous temporal bone to exclude any bony erosion which is a known complication of this infection.

2.6.6 Complications

External auditory meatus and canal stenosis. Chronic ear discharge.

2.6.7 Essential facts

Referral to otolaryngology should be considered after failure of initial course of topical antibiotics. Oral antibiotics are NOT recommended for otitis externa as they are ineffective and promote antibiotic resistance. Topical antibiotic penetration may be difficult due to copious discharge requiring microsuction.

2.7 Otitis media

2.7.1 Introduction

Serous otitis media

In this condition, fluid forms and collects in the middle ear behind the tympanic membrane due to acute or chronic nose, sinus, or throat infections causing inflammation and subsequent blockage of the Eustachian tube. This impairs its function of equalizing pressure in the middle ear cavity (see *Section 2.1*); as the air present within the middle ear is absorbed, no new air can enter the middle ear cavity to replace it (which happens during swallowing in a normal functioning Eustachian tube). This leads to the formation of negative pressure within this area, giving rise to inflammatory fluid formation in the middle ear cavity.

Acute otitis media

This is more common in children, where a viral or bacterial infection leads to acute inflammation of the middle ear. The patient complains of earache, blocked ear, and, in severe cases, mastoid tenderness due to involvement of mastoid air cells.

Chronic suppurative otitis media

This occurs when the initial infection was not adequately treated (possibly due to pathogen resistance or poor compliance), and the patient can present with acute or chronic ear discharge. The key is to identify if a cholesteatoma (see *Section 2.8*) is developing, which can cause local destruction of bone and ear infection.

2.7.2 Diagnosis

The diagnosis of otitis media (OM) is usually clinical; patients may present with a conductive hearing loss, earache, and/or discharge. Otoscopy (see *Section 1.2.1*) may demonstrate a fluid level with a gray or amber colored retracted tympanic membrane (**serous OM**) or a bulging, erythematous tympanic membrane (**acute OM**), or mucopurulent ear discharge with or without granulation tissue in the external auditory canal – white debris seen in the middle ear (**chronic suppurative OM with cholesteatoma**).

2.7.3 Investigations

Tympanogram (see *Section 1.5.2*): may be performed to evaluate for fluid in the middle ear (effusion) and determine if there is a perforation present. If discharge is present this could be sent for MC&S.

Imaging: CT or MRI may be required if there is a suspicion of cholesteatoma, which can lead to intracranial complications (see below); the patient may present with headache, fever, and pain / dizziness, and there may be suspicion of cholesteatoma.

2.7.4 Management

Serous otitis media

Medical: locally acting (minimally absorbed systemically) steroid nasal spray once or twice daily for 6–8 weeks may mitigate Eustachian tube dysfunction, which could be the cause of serous OM.

Nasal decongestant sprays can be used in acute cases. However, they should not be used for more than 3–5 days because they can lead to rebound nasal congestion complication, known as 'rhinitis medicamentosa'.

A combination of steroid and decongestant nasal drops/spray can be prescribed for a short period of up to 3–5 days. After that, a steroid-only spray can be used for a further 6–8 weeks.

In case of nasal, sinus, or throat infection a course of oral antibiotics should be recommended.

Otovent balloon inflation works as a form of exercise for the Eustachian tube. This can be done twice daily for 1–2 weeks, then once daily for 1 week, and then on an 'as and when required' basis. It significantly helps improve Eustachian tube function. The Valsalva maneuver may be performed several times a day for gentle exercise of the Eustachian tube.

Surgical: if a patient is not responding to medical treatment after 3 months then they may require myringotomy. In this procedure a small incision is made into the tympanic membrane to drain the fluid from the middle ear cavity and a pressure equalizing tube (PET or PE tube), also known as a grommet, is inserted under short general or local anesthesia.

After PE tube insertion, patients will need to be reviewed in outpatient clinic within 4 weeks and then followed up every 6 months until the PE tube comes out, usually after 6–24 months. Due to the improved ventilation, the middle ear mucosa will begin healing and start functioning properly, leading to expulsion of the PE tube. Hearing and pressure in the middle ear cavity will improve, which the patient will notice subjectively and which can be confirmed objectively by audiograms and tympanograms.

Some patients need reinsertion of PE tubes due to recurrence of persistent serous OM that does not respond to medical treatment.

Acute otitis media

Treatment is a course of antibiotics with steroid nasal spray and microsuction of ear discharge with culture and sensitivity, if there has been a perforation as a result of acute OM.

Chronic suppurative otitis media

With the presence of discharge, keeping the external ear canal as clear and dry as possible is crucial. This is performed via 'aural toilet', a technique using small caliber suction under the microscope. Obtaining specimens for culture and sensitivity may direct antimicrobial therapy. If there is discharge present, regular aural toilet and antibiotics are indicated. If the discharge does not resolve with these measures it may warrant hospital admission for intravenous antibiotic and further investigations.

As result of OM the patient can develop perforation of the eardrum (see *Section 2.9*).

2.7.5 Complications

Acute mastoiditis

This is infection and inflammation of the mastoid air cells; importantly, it involves pus formation and can cause bone necrosis. Due to antibiotic treatment for acute otitis media, complications are rare now; however, it is important to check for this – there will be tenderness on palpation of the mastoid process. It requires emergency ENT referral for intravenous antibiotic and further investigations. If this infection is because of cholesteatoma, the patient needs mastoid exploration to eradicate the disease.

A mastoid cavity is formed after mastoid exploration for the treatment of mastoiditis or the discharging ear, with or without cholesteatoma. Intra-operatively, the superior and posterior meatal bony walls are taken down, creating one large cavity. This cavity requires regular microsuction in the ENT clinic to prevent the accumulation of wax and debris, and to avoid secondary infection. The mastoid cavity often remains damp for up to 3 months post-operatively before drying up. Some mastoid cavities (up to 25%) will always discharge, usually with a mucoid discharge. However, the discharge may change to yellow-green when infected.

Other complications include:
* abscess formation (can be subperiosteal, extradural and even intracranial)
* meningitis
* labyrinthitis
* transverse or sigmoid sinus thrombosis
* cholesteatoma formation and its consequences (see *Section 2.8*)
* labyrinthine fistula
* ossicular erosion
* facial paralysis (lower motor neuron lesion).

2.7.6 Essential facts

Note that carcinoma of the nasopharynx can present with unilateral serous OM causing hearing loss. Nasopharyngeal cancer is most common in those of Asian (Chinese) ancestry. Thus it is important to examine post-nasal space, with nasal endoscopy or nasopharyngoscopy, in such patients to exclude nasopharyngeal pathology.

Acute-on-chronic otitis externa: if not treated or treatment fails, it can lead to meatal stenosis and malignant otitis externa (see *Section 2.1*).

2.8 Cholesteatoma

2.8.1 Introduction

A cholesteatoma is a non-cancerous growth of desquamated skin in the middle ear (the attic; see *Section 2.1*). It invades surrounding structures and can be one of two types; congenital or acquired (see below). It is usually a unilateral condition.

It is suggested that 1 in every 10 000 patients with ear discharge has a cholesteatoma, mainly the acquired form. Approximately 1 in 1000 patients referred to secondary care clinic with ear infection has a cholesteatoma.

Congenital cholesteatoma

This is thought to be the growth of normal skin at an abnormal place in the middle ear cavity which develops into a cholesteatoma. It is normally associated with an intact tympanic membrane, and usually occurs in children. It may occur in other locations, including the cerebellopontine angle.

Acquired cholesteatoma

This develops due to the failure of the mechanism regulating middle ear pressures.

If the Eustachian tube (see *Section 2.1*) does not function properly (e.g. in recurrent nose, sinus, throat, and ear infections where swelling of the tube will subsequently lead to its blockage), the middle ear pressure cannot be maintained and falls into negative pressure. This sucks in the tympanic membrane toward the middle ear cavity. This will create a small pocket behind, as it continues to be drawn inside and begins collecting desquamated skin from the surrounding area, which would normally be shed. This pocket grows at the expense of the middle ear and its structures (e.g. the ossicles) and progresses toward the inner ear, impacting on hearing and later balance.

2.8.2 Diagnosis

Patients may present with:
- recurrent ear infection with foul-smelling ear discharge
- gradual worsening of hearing
- tinnitus
- headache
- vertigo
- consequences of facial nerve impairment (e.g. unilateral facial droop; see *Section 2.20*).

On examination, there may be a unilateral facial droop present with associated weakness of the facial muscles (reflecting the extent of the mass) or tenderness on palpation of the mastoid process (indicative of complications; see *Section 2.8.6*). During otoscopy, the following may be seen:
- squamous debris in the external auditory canal and in the middle ear, particularly in the attic region

- perforation of the tympanic membrane
- a pearly white greasy mass (the cholesteatoma itself).

2.8.3 Causes

See *Section 2.7.1*.

2.8.4 Investigations

Ear swab: should be sent for C&S – *Pseudomonas* infection is usually responsible for the foul smell of the discharge.

Audiogram (see *Section 1.5.1*): this would show a conductive hearing loss.

CT scan of temporal bones: should be performed to check for extent of the disease in the surrounding structures.

2.8.5 Management

This condition requires surgical mastoid exploration to remove the cholesteatoma and diseased bone. In some cases, a second operation is required to improve hearing. Regular follow-up in ENT is advised, to monitor the ear cavity.

Non-surgical treatment is for patients who cannot undergo, or are not consenting to a general anesthetic; it is not first-line treatment. In such cases, treatment is with regular follow-up in otolaryngology with microsuction of the cholesteatoma which will prevent inward growth of the cholesteatoma and recurrent ear infection.

2.8.6 Complications

- Extensive middle ear infection with destruction of surrounding structures
- Acute mastoiditis (see *Section 2.7.5*)
- Brain abscess
- Meningitis.

2.8.7 Essential facts

Cholesteatoma or infection of the middle ear cavity is an **ENT emergency** and needs referral to ENT urgently for assessment and further treatment.

2.9 Perforation of the tympanic membrane

2.9.1 Introduction

The tympanic membrane (also known as the eardrum see *Section 2.1*) is an integral component of the hearing pathway. This tough and flexible membrane is approximately 0.1 mm thick and 14 mg in weight.

2.9.2 Diagnosis

The patient may present with the following symptoms if it is an acute perforation:
- severe otalgia and, conversely, patients may experience severe pain which is resolved at the time of the perforation
- tinnitus
- acute hearing loss up to 40 dB depending on the size and location of the perforation.

Chronic perforation may present with:
- recurrent ear infections
- chronic ear drainage.

Both are due to getting water in the ear or recurring upper respiratory tract infections. With chronic ear drainage, recurrent infections can change the lining of the middle ear and mastoid cavity. These then produce excessive mucoid drainage which frequently becomes infected and leads to more chronic drainage.

On examination, the perforation will be visible on otoscopy.

2.9.3 Causes

The most common causes of perforation of the tympanic membrane include:
- trauma (accidental or operative); a frequent cause is Q-tips
- infection (OM; see *Section 2.7*).

2.9.4 Investigations

An audiogram (see *Section 1.5.1*) should be performed for cases of perforation. This would be required at both initial presentation and follow-up.

A tympanogram will show no pressure in the middle ear cavity, as the perforation does not allow pressure to build. Additionally, there will be a large ear canal volume because the tympanogram measures the volume of the external canal and the middle ear cavity.

2.9.5 Management

A small perforation not causing any symptoms (see above) does not require treatment, because it will generally heal spontaneously.

In acute traumatic perforation, the patient should be treated conservatively with water avoidance and no ear drops, and reviewed after 6 weeks. In a large number of patients (up to 94% in some studies), the perforation is healed.

In the case of symptomatic perforation that cannot be managed in this way, the affected discharging ear will require myringoplasty or tympanoplasty as the surgical procedures of choice. Note that the aims of this surgery are to dry the ear and to prevent ear infection. This surgery does not aim to improve hearing; if hearing improves as a result of this surgery, this is an added bonus.

In cases where there is damage to the ossicles, ossiculoplasty can also be performed to try to improve hearing.

2.9.6 Essential facts

These patients need to be referred to specialist ENT clinics for care.

2.10 Otosclerosis

2.10.1 Introduction

Otosclerosis most commonly affects Caucasians and females and usually presents before the age of 30. This disease is genetic (autosomal dominant); however, sporadic cases are also seen.

It is due to otospongiosis of the footplate of the stapes – there is thickening of the bone where the footplate of the stapes sits over the oval window (see *Section 2.1*); this is normally a thin tough elastic ring called annular ligament. The stapes becomes rigid and sound vibrations cannot pass freely from the oval window to the inner ear, preventing sound from reaching the cochlea. This condition progresses slowly until the footplate of the stapes is completely fixed and hearing is severely affected. This condition should be considered in all patients presenting with hearing loss (conductive) under the age of 40 and with a family history of early hearing loss.

2.10.2 Diagnosis

It is characterized by conductive hearing loss and tinnitus, with or without vertigo. There are no specific findings on examination of the tympanic membrane.

This disease is usually bilateral; however, both ears may not be affected at the same time. Some individuals experience only unilateral disease.

2.10.3 Causes

There has been no cause identified for this pathology, other than the genetic preponderance.

2.10.4 Investigations

Tuning fork test (see *Section 1.4.2*): Weber will be heard better on the affected side and the Rinne test will show bone conduction better than air conduction on the affected side.

Audiogram (see *Section 1.5.1*): this will show results consistent with conductive hearing loss on the affected side (an air–bone gap will be seen). *Figure 2.3* shows an audiogram suggestive of this.

Tympanogram: this will show normal pressure in the middle ear cavity.

MRI petrous temporal bone: this can be used to confirm the otospongiosis.

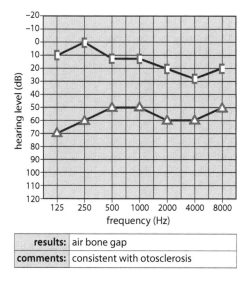

results:	air bone gap
comments:	consistent with otosclerosis

Figure 2.3 Audiogram consistent with otosclerosis. The squares show bone conduction and the triangles air conduction.

2.10.5 Management

Surgery (stapedectomy) is the treatment of choice in young patients. A prosthesis is used to bypass the otospongiosis of footplate of the stapes as it is not possible to remove the regrowth of new bone. Post-operatively the patient will require six-monthly follow-up in ENT for two years, with audiogram.

Conservative treatment is with a hearing aid; this is usually recommended to patients in whom surgery is contraindicated or which is undesirable to the patient. Surgical treatment is also not recommended if the patient only has one ear as there is a minute chance of dead ear.

2.10.6 Complications

If left untreated the hearing loss gradually worsens; a significant number of patients state that the hearing loss stabilizes at moderate to severe levels of hearing loss. However, a small percentage of patients become profoundly deaf.

Nerve damage intra-operatively

The chorda tympani nerve, which carries taste fibers from the anterior third of the tongue, passes through the eardrum on its way to join the facial nerve. This nerve can be damaged or bruised during stapedectomy, and the patient's sense of taste can be damaged or altered on the operated side. The patient may complain of a metallic taste in the mouth which usually resolves by itself; however, it may take many months.

Profound deafness post-surgery

The major risk of the surgery is that in a very small percentage of patients, some inner ear changes occur (with no apparent reason seen) which can lead to disabling symptoms of profound deafness, tinnitus and vertigo. However, surgery transforms the individual's life through the return of hearing to normal levels.

2.10.7 Essential facts

In some women, progression of hearing loss has been seen to be associated with pregnancy, either appearing during a pregnancy or worsening soon after giving birth. It appears that the hormonal changes of pregnancy speed up the process of fixation of the footplate of the stapes. Hearing deteriorates quickly over the nine months of pregnancy.

If you suspect this condition, the patient requires referral to otolaryngology/an otologist. A typical case is that of a young woman with a history of hearing loss and a family history of hearing loss at an early age. If it is associated with pregnancy, this diagnosis should be high on the list of differentials.

2.11 Acoustic neuroma

2.11.1 Introduction

Acoustic neuroma, also known as vestibular schwannoma, is a benign non-cancerous growth. It is a nerve sheath growth affecting the superior vestibular nerve within the internal auditory meatus. It is a slow-growing tumor and the age of presentation is usually between 40 and 60 years.

2.11.2 Diagnosis

The most common symptom is unilateral, and usually progressive, hearing loss associated with tinnitus and occasionally vertigo. Expansion of the growth in the cerebellopontine angle can present with ataxia and unsteadiness.

On examination, the ear will appear normal; however, in severe cases cranial nerve examination or cerebellar examination may indicate the presence of complications due to involvement of surrounding cranial nerves (VII) or brain structures.

2.11.3 Investigations

Imaging: MRI scan of internal auditory canal with gadolinium contrast is the *gold standard* investigation for this condition.

Stapedial reflex: this reflex is absent in about 90% of patients. It is an involuntary muscle contraction that occurs in the middle ear muscles in response to high intensity sound stimuli, in order to protect the ear from loud noise damage. The audiologist can evaluate this with the tympanogram.

Audiogram: this test (see *Section 1.5.1*) will demonstrate an asymmetrical hearing loss.

2.11.4 Management

In cases where there is small intracanalicular growth with minimal to no symptoms, regular follow-up with yearly MRI scan of the internal auditory canal is recommended.

Surgical excision in expert hands carries good results, but there is still a risk of complete hearing loss in some patients. The surgical decision is usually based on the age and health of the patient in addition to their desire for surgical intervention which may result in complete hearing loss. With a strong suspicion of acoustic neuroma, the patient should be referred to a neurotologist.

Radiotherapy is recommended in some patients where surgery is not possible.

Conservative treatment is usually recommended in elderly patients with no complications, as it is a slow-growing lesion.

2.11.5 Essential facts

Unilateral hearing loss with tinnitus in the affected ear only is an **ENT emergency**. In primary care, if such a patient is seen with no obvious cause for hearing loss (see *Section 2.2*) referral to otolaryngology is required for further investigations and diagnosis. Definitive treatment of acoustic neuroma requires evaluation by a neurotologist.

2.12 The draining ear

2.12.1 Introduction

Any type of secretion from the ear is called otorrhea, irrespective of cause.
It can be unilateral or bilateral. It is almost always associated with other symptoms
(see *Section 1.1*).

2.12.2 Diagnosis

The history will be important in narrowing the list of differentials; however, a thorough
examination of the ear under microscope, with microsuction of the discharge, will
be very helpful. Some distinguishing characteristics of the discharge may be key in
determining the cause.

- Cheesy-looking discharge with white or black spores in it
  - likely fungal
- Yellow-green discharge, sometimes with streaks of blood in it
  - likely acute or acute on chronic infection
- Clear discharge; if this is present
  - immediately evaluate for CSF (see below), particularly if there is a history of
    trauma or any possibility of base of skull fractures, as well as
  - checking for other signs of CSF leak.

2.12.3 Causes

Most common	Eczema, psoriasis or dermatitis of the external auditory canal
	Fungal or bacterial otitis externa (see *Section 2.6*)
	Furuncle in the external auditory canal (see *Section 2.22*)
	Mastoiditis (see *Section 2.7.5*)
	OM +/– cholesteatoma formation (see *Section 2.7*)
	Perforation of tympanic membrane (see *Section 2.9*)
	Trauma to external, middle or inner ear or base of skull fracture
Least common	Radionecrosis of external auditory canal

2.12.4 Investigations

Ear swab: a swab of the discharge should be sent to the laboratory for C&S. On
average preliminary results should be available within 48 hours; however, full
sensitivities may take up to 5 days (please check your lab for specific times).

Glucose test: in cases of clear ear discharge, test for glucose to exclude a CSF leak.

Imaging: MRI scan of internal auditory canal is the modality of choice in suspected cholesteatoma; however, if there are contraindications to having an MRI scan (see *Section 1.7.1*), consider a CT scan instead. If there is difficulty with insurance co-pays, a CT of the temporal bone is acceptable as evaluation of possible cholesteatoma.

2.12.5 Management

This should be directed to the individual cause (see *Section 2.2* for individual sections).

Steroid ear drops for *eczema* and for other *non-infective, inflammatory skin* conditions should be advised for use for only 1–2 weeks initially, then under supervision of the clinician as needed.

A suspected cholesteatoma (see *Section 2.8*) requires surgical exploration of the middle ear and mastoid cavity, and therefore needs to be excluded urgently when reviewing ear discharge; refer to ENT.

2.12.6 Complications

These are particular to the underlying cause of the otorrhea. They can be extensive and serious and therefore need to be actively looked for and explored. Complications can range from perforation of the tympanic membrane to intracranial abscess. Please check individual sections for further details.

2.12.7 Essential facts

A discharging ear with vertigo / unsteadiness and/or tinnitus with or without facial weakness is an **ENT emergency** with the possible diagnosis of cholesteatoma with complications (see *Section 2.8*).

Antibiotic or antifungal ear drops in combination with steroids are indicated in bacterial or fungal infection for 2–3 weeks. Advice should also be given regarding precautions against water entering the ear.

Recurrent ear discharge not resolved with treatment at primary care level with antibiotic ear drops needs referral to specialist care ENT clinic, where treatment should consist of gentle regular ear toilet (microsuction of ear discharge under microscope) and further evaluation.

2.13 Earache

2.13.1 Introduction

Otalgia, also known as earache or pain in the ear, is a common presentation in primary care clinic. It can affect any age group. Earache can be due to local causes or be referred pain.

Local causes include diseases of the pinna, external auditory meatus, external auditory canal, tympanic membrane, middle ear, mastoid, and inner ear.

The ear has a rich nerve supply including facial, trigeminal, vagus, and glossopharyngeal nerves. Below are common sites of **referred pain**:
*   TMJ
*   teeth / dental (via fifth cranial nerve, mandibular division)
*   tongue (via glossopharyngeal nerve), floor of mouth, submandibular or parotid glands (via fifth cranial nerve, mandibular division)
*   tonsil (via the glossopharyngeal nerve)
*   larynx and pharynx
*   cervical spine.

2.13.2 Diagnosis

Clinical assessment (see *Sections 1.1* and *1.2*) should be able to identify any ENT pathology which may be causing earache. Inspection is an important aspect of earache assessment, because if vesicles are seen in the external auditory meatus or on the tympanic membrane, this would be consistent with Ramsay Hunt syndrome (herpes virus affecting the geniculate ganglion – known to be especially painful; see *Section 2.19*).

In light of the rich nerve supply of the ear it is important to review referred pain sites (above) when assessing for earache, especially as malignant diseases of the tongue, larynx and hypopharynx often present with earache. Resist the kneejerk temptation to diagnose all ear pain as otitis (externa or media).

Be sure to examine the TMJ; in severe TMJ disease the joint may be tender on palpation, and otoscopic examination of the ear may be just as painful (the otoscope will press on the joint during examination). In the history, the patient may experience jaw 'clicking' when they open their mouth. Some people complain of severe earache when they lie on the affected side, with the pain even waking them up at night.

2.13.3 Causes

Below are some of the most common causes; see individual sections (listed in *Section 2.2*) for specific management.
*   Furuncle of the ear
*   OM (serous) and (acute)

- Otitis externa (acute)
- Mastoiditis
- Wax
- Foreign body in the ear
- Ramsay Hunt syndrome
- Referred ear pain (see above).

Other causes, not uncommon, of referred earache are glossopharyngeal neuralgia and elongated styloid process, known as Eagle syndrome. These would be diagnosed and require specialist management.

2.13.4 Investigations

Audiogram (see *Section 1.5.1*) and **tympanogram** (see *Section 1.5.2*): these are helpful in exploring earache secondary to an ear pathology.

If the ear appears normal on examination and the above-mentioned hearing tests are within normal limits, then referred earache needs to be explored again – especially as **head and neck cancers can also present with earache**.

2.13.5 Essential facts

Tonsillectomy, especially within the first 10 days post-operatively, is a significant cause of earache.

For cervical spine lesions (especially C2 and C3) presenting as earache, this pain is often worse at night; neck support often provides relief.

2.14 Vertigo and dizziness

2.14.1 Introduction

This disabling symptom cannot be expressed with enough gravity through mere words. Dizziness is used by patients to describe subjective sensations of imbalance, unsteadiness, or rotational movement. It is a symptom, not a disease, and usually understood as the feeling of movement when there is no movement. It helps the diagnostic process if this concept is split into three distinct streams: **vertigo**, **imbalance**, and **syncope**, based on etiologies and subjective feelings.

Vertigo originates from dysfunction of the vestibular system and its connections (i.e. the balance system). Pathologies can be split into peripheral (benign paroxysmal positional vertigo (see *Section 2.15*), labyrinthitis (see *Section 2.16*), Ménière's disease (see *Section 2.17*)) and central causes (migraine (also vestibular migraine), multiple sclerosis, or vertebrobasilar insufficiency).

- Rotational vertigo is of vestibular origin, whereas non-rotational vertigo implies disturbance outside the ear.
- Generally vertigo is thoroughly evaluated prior to treatment. Phenothiazines and anticholinergic medications cause significant side-effects. Patients seen in the ED, Urgent or Primary care are frequently given meclizine for symptomatic relief.
- True vertigo, that is continuous for a few days without any asymptomatic periods, warrants referral to hospital to identify cardiac or neurological pathology. Although a rarer presentation, stroke can occur in the brainstem and involve the vestibular nuclei, hence thorough assessment is required to exclude potentially life-threatening causes.

Vertigo is always associated with **imbalance** but imbalance is not always due to vertigo. Imbalance is usually due to extra-aural causes such as cardiovascular, metabolic, musculoskeletal, ocular diseases, or stress. These are not discussed in further detail in this book.

Syncope is related to the sensation of losing consciousness and again is not related to the balance system directly. Causes of this are cardiovascular, hematological, secondary to medications, or vasovagal.

2.14.2 Causes

The most important tool in the assessment of such a symptom is taking a complete history to establish which diagnostic stream (see above) needs to be investigated. Examination needs to include ENT, cardiovascular, neurological (including cerebellar, central and peripheral nervous system), and vision.

If it has been established that the patient is suffering from vertigo then see *Section 2.2* on how to manage each individual cause. Note that vertigo associated with new onset deafness and/or tinnitus, especially unilateral, is an **ENT emergency** and needs urgent ENT referral.

It is estimated that approximately 26% of dizziness patients presenting to primary care are secondary to psychological causes and input by psychology or psychiatry is indicated.

2.14.3 Essential facts

The impact on quality of life of this symptom cannot be underestimated and a significant number of patients may withdraw from activities and show avoidance behavior out of fear. Reassurance and support is key not only psychologically but because it will support the compensatory mechanisms.

Migrainous vertigo should be treated along the migraine pathway, including possible neurological evaluation.

2.15 Benign paroxysmal positional vertigo

2.15.1 Introduction

Benign paroxysmal positional vertigo (BPPV) occurs after a head injury or ear infection, such as vestibular neuronitis or labyrinthitis. But most commonly it is idiopathic and occurs spontaneously. The balance apparatus of the ear consists of semicircular canals and the otolith organ containing otolith (see *Section 2.1*) and is responsible for our sense of gravity. If for any reason these pieces of calcium dislodge into the semicircular canal, they can then cause this off-balance feeling.

2.15.2 Diagnosis

Patients will report intermittent episodes of feeling off-balance associated with particular head movements. This sensation lasts from seconds to minutes without hearing loss or tinnitus. Activities which may trigger an episode include getting in and out of bed, looking upward (top-shelf vertigo), tying shoe laces or bending to pick something up from the ground.

On examination, if the Dix–Hallpike test reproduces the patient's symptoms together with the presence of rotatory nystagmus, this supports the diagnosis of BPPV. This test must be used with caution in those with neck pathology.

Nystagmus characteristically starts after a latency of a few seconds and fatigues on repetition.

2.15.3 Causes

Most common	Idiopathic
	Trauma to the head
	Prolonged extension of the neck for any reason, e.g. sleeping in an awkward position
Least common	Migraine

2.15.4 Management

The treatment of choice for BPPV sufferers should be the Epley maneuver; it can be effective in 80% of cases.
- This maneuver will reposition the otoliths in the semicircular canal and the patient's symptoms should improve within a week.

- Post-procedure the patient should be followed up in four weeks to confirm resolution.
- This is a specialist test and should not be performed in primary care until a specially trained professional is available; otherwise refer to ENT.
- Some patients need a repeat Epley maneuver to attain complete recovery.

This condition is generally self-limiting and resolves spontaneously within a few months.

Supportive advice is key to ensure patients remain mobile and do not start withdrawing from their regular activities; this could hinder the compensatory mechanism which itself can aid recovery. In fact, instructing the patient about exercises recreating the symptoms can help to extinguish the symptoms.

2.16 Labyrinthitis

2.16.1 Introduction

Labyrinthitis is one of the most common causes of vertigo. It is usually viral in origin; however, it can also be bacterial. This is more common when caused by cholesteatoma in a chronically discharging ear or in cases of operative trauma.

2.16.2 Diagnosis

The patient describes sudden onset disabling vertigo associated with tinnitus, although hearing is usually normal. However, some patients describe 'dull' hearing.

Depending on the cause of the disease (see below) there may be a history of chronic ear discharge. On examination, there may also be signs of complications of the underlying disease, e.g. facial nerve weakness (see *Section 2.8*).

On examination during an acute attack there may be nystagmus (unidirectional and horizontal, with the fast phase towards the side of lesion initially and then later towards the unaffected ear).

2.16.3 Causes

Most common → Least common	
	Viral labyrinthitis
	Bacterial labyrinthitis
	Drugs, either due to direct ototoxicity or central effects, e.g. aminoglycosides (gentamicin), diuretics, co-trimoxazole, and metronidazole therapy
	Syphilis involvement of balance apparatus
	Idiopathic

2.16.4 Management

Labyrinthitis is an acute emergency; patients can be given symptomatic treatment of anti-emetic and vestibular sedatives (antihistamines, benzodiazepines, and anticholinergics). It is important that patients remain mobile and do not withdraw completely from activities as this may hinder compensatory mechanisms for recovery.

Generally, patients should be referred to ENT for confirmation of diagnosis and supportive therapy.

Infection

If viral in origin, an infection should resolve on its own within a few weeks or months. The patient will need symptomatic treatment for dizziness and/or nausea. If the infection is bacterial in origin, the patient will need antibiotics to treat the causative infection.

Trauma

This requires supportive therapy and the patient should be assessed and treated for fracture.

Cholesteatoma

See *Section 2.8* for treatment, which includes mastoid exploration.

2.17 Ménière's disease

2.17.1 Introduction

This is a condition caused by an imbalance within the endolymphatic system in the inner ear, leading to episodic tinnitus, vertigo and hearing loss. It is estimated to affect both sexes equally and commonly occurs in those aged 40–60 years. It is considered a diagnosis of exclusion, based on history and physical examination, along with an audiogram which typically shows low frequency sensorineural hearing loss in the affected ear.

2.17.2 Diagnosis

Patients suffer from intermittent vertigo, episodes which are unpredictable and can last from many minutes to hours, associated with unilateral sensorineural hearing loss, aural fullness, tinnitus, sound distortion, or diplacusis. It is a unilateral disease, but rarely presents bilaterally. There may also be nausea, with or without vomiting.

Migraine was once thought to be one of the most common causes of dizziness. However, in a migraine, the severe dizziness and vomiting may be associated with headache (although not always), and it is not usually associated with hearing deficit or tinnitus.

On examination, it is important to exclude causes of syncope or other neurological conditions (e.g. stroke / transient ischemic attack or multiple sclerosis). In a central lesion during vertigo, there is an immediate onset of nystagmus unaffected by gaze fixation and the patient rarely feels nauseated. The patient may also have other cerebellar signs on clinical examination.

Unterberger test

- The patient is asked to close their eyes and march on the spot with their arms held out in front of them.
- The side that drifts from the center is suggestive of the side of vestibular dysfunction.

Romberg's test

- This requires that the patient stand with their arms and legs together, initially with their eyes open then shut.
- With intact vision and vestibular systems, the patient will be able to maintain their balance with their eyes open. As they shut their eyes, if there is impairment of proprioception, the patient will open their eyes to avoid losing their balance.
- As there is a risk of the patient losing their balance if they close their eyes, the examiner should remain close by and reassure the patient of this.

2.17.3 Causes

Ménière's disease is a disease of idiopathic causation; however, Ménière's syndrome (which is much rarer) is thought to be secondary to endocrine abnormalities, trauma, parasitic infections, hyperlipidemia, or medications. Note that in the US the terms Ménière's disease and Ménière's syndrome may be used interchangeably.

2.17.4 Investigations

Audiogram: in this disease, an audiogram (see *Section 1.5.1* for further details) is essential and may show evidence of a sensorineural hearing loss. Classically this loss is described as low frequency (see *Figure 2.4*). A fluctuating sensorineural loss shown on consecutive audiograms over a period of time and with an appropriate history provides good evidence for an accurate diagnosis.

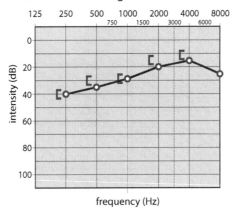

Figure 2.4 Audiogram typical of Ménière's disease.

Tympanogram: used to investigate the pressure in the middle ear (see *Section 1.5.2*).

Caloric test: before the test the patient should be warned that it can cause dizziness (see *Section 1.6.1*). This test may show impaired vestibular function and will also show the presence of canal paralysis, which will be elicited as it causes less nystagmus.

Electronystagmogram: this is performed to evaluate balance function (see *Section 1.6.2*).

Equi test: this test (a brand name for posturography, see *Section 1.6.3*) is used to explore how impaired balance impacts the patient's ability to carry out day-to-day activities.

Radiology: an MRI scan of the internal auditory canal should be done to exclude acoustic neuroma or cerebellopontine angle lesion. Additionally, MRI is now able to display endolymphatic hydrops and may confirm diagnostically difficult cases.

Blood tests: these should be advised if the diagnosis is in doubt or according to the merit of the disease (especially if considering Ménière's syndrome or other systemic conditions). Common tests include CBC, CMP, fasting blood sugar level, lipid profile, and autoimmune screen (ANA (antinuclear antibody), ANCA, rheumatoid factor).

2.17.5 Management

Acute attack

An acute attack of Ménière's disease is an **ENT emergency** and the patient needs to be referred to the ED for management. Some patients require hospital admission for the treatment which includes anti-emetic, betahistine or vasodilators, and, if needed, intravenous fluids for vomiting and dehydration.

When the patient is more stable they will require audiograms which will show low frequency mixed hearing loss. During the acute stage of an attack, the patient feels that their hearing is significantly decreased and as the acute stage passes, the hearing improves. However, it does not revert to the previous normal stage. With the passage of time, due to repeated episodes of Ménière's disease, the patient experiences long-term hearing loss.

Short-term measures

In the US, immediate care generally consists of anti-emetics and referral to ENT. Also recommended is low CATS (caffeine, alcohol, tobacco and sodium (or salt)) diet.

Gentle neck exercises are also beneficial in some patients, but these should be used with caution if neck pathology is present.

The patient should be referred to Physical Therapy for rehabilitation.

Long-term treatments

Vestibular rehabilitation is considered the mainstay of treatment for vertigo as it targets the formation of adequate compensatory mechanisms to be achieved from the working vestibule and other balance organs, chiefly the eyes and proprioception.

The potassium-sparing diuretic combination of hydrochlorothiazide and triamterene 25/37.5 is generally safe and effective to control the symptoms of Ménière's syndrome/disease. Medical management is preferred in this condition as, over time, there appears to be a 'burnout' of the condition.

Surgery is mainly used for Ménière's disease where medical treatment has failed. It may be divided into hearing preserving surgery, such as saccus decompression and vestibular neuronectomy, or hearing destructive surgery, such as labyrinthectomy. Injection of aminoglycosides in the round window is another effective option.

2.17.6 Essential facts

When taking the history it is very important to clearly ascertain the original onset of the problem, associated symptoms, and progression of the disease.

Drivers' licensing laws vary by state for patients with vertigo, but the appropriate agency may need to be notified about the condition and any treatment being received for it.

2.18 Tinnitus

2.18.1 Introduction

Tinnitus is the perception by the patient of sound which is produced without stimulation from the external environment. It can be unilateral or bilateral in the ears, continuous or intermittent. The intensity and frequency of these sounds can vary. These sounds have been proven to impact on patients' quality of life, especially on their sleep. Patients hear these sounds as a result of changes in the auditory pathway.

These sounds are usually described as 'crickets', ringing or a whooshing sound in a low or high tone. In some patients it is described as pulsatile. Tinnitus is subjective; however, very rarely it can be objective, such as in the case where the other person can hear what the patient perceives – this occurs when it is vascular in nature, or caused by a muscle spasm.

2.18.2 Causes

Most common	Loud noise exposure
	Acute perforation of tympanic membrane
	Serous OM
	Eustachian tube dysfunction
	Viral upper respiratory tract infection
	Hearing loss
Least common	Anxiety / stress
	Trauma to the head
	Otosclerosis
	Acoustic neuroma
	Ramsay Hunt syndrome

2.18.3 Investigations

Audiogram: used to investigate any hearing loss (see *Section 1.5.1*).

Tympanogram: used to evaluate the health of the tympanic membrane and will also identify any effusions (see *Section 1.5.2*).

Imaging: an MRI scan of internal auditory canal is used to exclude an acoustic neuroma, especially when the tinnitus is unilateral.

2.18.4 Management

Management consists of treating the underlying disease; see *Section 2.2* to be directed to disease-specific management.

Hearing aids can be prescribed for those who have associated hearing loss. Often restoration of hearing with hearing aids overcomes tinnitus by allowing the brain threshold of hearing to be reset, and so the tinnitus is no longer heard.

A bedside radio or pillow radio can help patients go to sleep, in cases where tinnitus is impairing their sleep. Numerous supplements, primarily vitamins, mineral and herbal supplements are available over the counter which purport to help relieve the symptoms of tinnitus, though there isn't a strong evidence base for their efficacy.

A white noise generator is useful for patients with minimal or no hearing loss. A combination of hearing aid and white noise generator is advised for a patient suffering from both hearing loss and tinnitus.

When there is no obvious cause identified, there are no positive findings, the tinnitus is not unilateral, and the disease is not affecting the patient's quality of life, treatment is through reassurance.

Most tinnitus fades into insignificance and becomes less disturbing with the passage of time due to natural compensation and a sense of reassurance that nothing pathological is causing the tinnitus. A small percentage of patients do show good signs of recovery after tinnitus counseling. In very severe cases, rarely, measures such as antidepressant therapy and destruction of the auditory apparatus are advised.

2.18.5 Essential facts

If the patient describes vascular tinnitus then you should examine for a carotid bruit. In fact, for objective pulsatile tinnitus, angiography may be necessary if a specific vascular lesion is suspected.

Sudden onset **unilateral** tinnitus, with or without dizziness or hearing loss and negative acute ear, nose, and throat infection on examination is an **ENT emergency** and should be referred to ENT for urgent investigation.

2.19 Presbycusis

2.19.1 Introduction

This is a progressive degeneration of the auditory system due to gradual loss of the hair cells in the organ of Corti (see *Section 2.1*) which are responsible for transmitting sound in electrical form to the brain. This is associated with aging and leads to hearing impairment with reduced acuteness in hearing, referred to as decreased speech discrimination.

Loss of these hair cells is worse at the base of cochlea which deals with high frequencies, which are very important for hearing in the presence of background noise. Consequently, the hearing loss associated with presbycusis is initially seen at higher frequencies and is most notable in loud environments with ample background noise.

2.19.2 Diagnosis

It is important to ask about onset of hearing loss, history of loud noise exposure, any history of trauma or acute ENT infections. In general, patients present with a gradual decrease in their hearing and/or tinnitus. They or their family may note that speech discrimination is significantly affected regardless of the loudness of the sound because the patient's ear loses its ability to differentiate between very similar sounds. Typically, the patient will note initial difficulty in crowded noisy settings such as social gatherings or restaurants.

Examination is normally unremarkable; however, it is essential to rule out any other cause of the patient's presenting symptoms.

2.19.3 Investigations

Audiogram: classically shows a high frequency sensorineural hearing loss in both ears (see *Section 1.5.1*).

2.19.4 Management

There are no treatments to reverse the condition. However, patients can usually be referred to audiology to be assessed for suitability for a hearing aid, with or without lip reading therapy.

2.20 Facial paralysis

2.20.1 Introduction

The facial nerve is the seventh cranial nerve (see *Figure 2.5*) and supplies the muscles of facial expression, parasympathetic efferents to the lacrimal gland and submandibular gland, and taste afferents from the anterior two-thirds of the tongue. The upper face has a dual innervation from both hemispheres of brain, whereas lower facial muscles are supplied by the contralateral hemisphere only. It is important to note that a number of ear pathologies can cause this symptom.

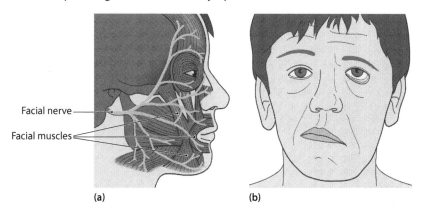

Facial nerve

Facial muscles

(a)   (b)

Figure 2.5 (a) Facial nerve, together with its muscle nerve supply; (b) presentation of facial paralysis.
Part (b) reproduced from *Applied Knowledge Test for the MRCGP*, fourth edition, © Scion Publishing Ltd, 2017.

2.20.2 Diagnosis

Patients will present with numbness or weakness of the facial muscles, watering of the eye with a drooping of the eyelid, difficulty articulating speech, and taste disturbance. Depending on the cause of the paralysis, patients may have ear discharge or a reduction in their hearing.

On examination, there will be flattening of the nasolabial fold, hyperesthesia in the distribution of trigeminal nerve, and hyperacusis.

2.20.3 Causes

Most common	Bell's palsy	• This is an acute lower motor neuron lesion of unknown cause. • Accounts for more than 35% of facial paralysis cases. • Diagnosis depends on exclusion of other causes.
	Ramsay Hunt syndrome	• Caused by herpes zoster oticus infection of facial nerve. It is known to be more painful than Bell's palsy, which is generally painless. • Incidence rate is 7%. • Classically, there is an erythematous vesicular rash of the skin of the ear canal, auricle, and mucous membrane of the oropharynx.
	Head trauma involving squamous or petrous part of the temporal bone	Accidental trauma or surgical intervention can cause facial palsy. It is very important to know the extent of the injury as soon as possible. Despite this, chances of full recovery are not very high.
	Serous OM	This can lead to facial palsy if there is a dehiscence of the facial canal.
	Chronic suppurative OM with complications	This is a combination of facial palsy in the context of a chronically discharging ear, probably with cholesteatoma formation.
	Malignant otitis externa	This is usually seen in older diabetic patients with recurrent ear infections and is associated with *Pseudomonas* infections.
	Malignant growth in the ear	A malignancy of the external auditory canal, middle ear and that of the parotid gland can involve the facial nerve at varying points in its course.
Least common	Systemic diseases	For example, multiple sclerosis, brainstem infarction, cerebellopontine angle lesions, poliomyelitis.

2.20.4 Investigations

Audiogram: used to investigate the extent and quality of hearing loss (see *Section 1.5.1*).

Tympanogram: used to evaluate the health of the tympanic membrane and will also identify any effusions (see *Section 1.5.2*) or perforations not visible.

Imaging: MRI or CT of the petrous temporal bone (preferably MRI if no contraindications) is used to identify any mass lesion or dehiscence of the facial nerve in its canal.

Blood tests: request the following: CBC, CMP, TFTs, ESR, viral titers, syphilis serology and FTA absorption, blood sugar levels.

Lacrimation test: this test will show reduced flow of tears on the ipsilateral side of the facial paralysis. Similarly the **taste test** will delineate the taste impairment and, depending upon the extent of the impairment, reflect the severity of the palsy.

Electrodiagnostic tests: used to assess the severity of paralysis.

2.20.5 Management

The aim of the treatment for facial nerve paralysis is to alleviate the disability and to provide the nerve with the best chance of recovery.

Eye care is mandatory in order to prevent corneal ulceration; this involves artificial tears to be used 4–5 times a day and an eye patch to be worn at night. Ophthalmology advice should also be sought.

Active treatment is indicated in patients who are seen within 24 hours of the onset of symptoms and a short course of oral steroids can be commenced, provided there are no contraindications in the patient's medical history (they should be avoided in pulmonary tuberculosis, glaucoma, peptic ulcer, diabetes, pregnancy, and psychosis). Antiviral medication is used in the early stages of viral infections. Steroids are not recommended in this condition as they can lead to encephalitis.

Cases of **serous OM** (see *Section 2.7* for further details) should be treated conservatively initially. However, in resistant cases myringotomy and/or PE tube insertion is advocated.

Definitive surgery is recommended in cases of **cholesteatoma** (see *Section 2.8* for further details).

Idiopathic Bell's palsy begins to improve within 2 to 3 weeks, with 35–50% of people making a full recovery over a period of months. Prednisolone is effective if started within 72 hours of onset of symptoms. However, the palsy can recur in 12% of patients and is more common on the contralateral side.

Recurrence is very uncommon in **Ramsay Hunt syndrome**; however, recovery is not complete in the majority of the cases.

2.20.6 Essential facts

Any patient seen at primary care level with facial nerve weakness should be referred to an ENT clinic for further investigation and treatment. If the forehead is unaffected on examination, this suggests an upper motor neuron lesion, which needs neurological assessment and review.

If the nerve is suddenly damaged, no electrical test will show any abnormality until the peripheral part of the nerve has degenerated to the region where the test stimulus is applied.

Brainstem lesions will produce weakness of the facial muscle with no loss of taste and lacrimation.

Sometimes weakness of the abducent nerve is also present and this can cause diplopia due to the weakness of the lateral rectus muscle.

Loss of lacrimation and taste from the anterior third of the tongue alone, suggests a lesion between the brainstem and geniculate ganglion. Facial weakness with loss of taste but normal lacrimation indicates a lesion between the geniculate ganglion and the origin of the chorda tympani. If both taste and lacrimation are present, the lesion is peripheral to the stylomastoid foramen.

2.21 Foreign body in the ear

2.21.1 Introduction

Patients presenting with a foreign body in the ear are mostly young children, patients with chronic behavioral health illness or people who have been cleaning their ear with Q-tips. Common foreign bodies found include Q-tips, beads, pieces of building blocks, tissue paper or dead insects such as flies and cockroaches.

2.21.2 Diagnosis

Foreign bodies can be found accidentally by parents or caregivers, or patients themselves may complain of earache, irritation in the ear or ear discharge. Hearing may be affected if the external auditory canal is obstructed.

The foreign body should be visible in the external auditory meatus or canal, either with the naked eye or via otoscopy.

2.21.3 Management

Although foreign bodies are occasionally (rarely) successfully removed in the primary care setting, the ENT clinic is usually most appropriate. Children may require anesthesia for removal of a foreign body from the external auditory canal. It usually comes out at the first attempt with appropriate equipment. Unsuccessful attempts can push the foreign body further into the ear canal and can cause injury to the external auditory canal or tympanic membrane. Such foreign bodies need removal under a short general anesthetic in expert hands.

2.21.4 Essential facts

At primary care clinic, team members should not attempt to remove foreign bodies, irrespective of how easy it may appear to be, especially in children. This is because children may move suddenly which can traumatize the ear canal or push the foreign body deep into the canal, where it can damage the tympanic membrane.

2.22 Furuncle in the external auditory canal

2.22.1 Introduction

This is an infection, commonly by *Staphylococcus aureus*, of a hair follicle within the external auditory canal.

2.22.2 Diagnosis

Pain is significant, sometimes causing the patient to be unable to open their jaw. Even holding the pinna to examine the ear is very painful for the patient. Hearing loss and ear discharge can be present, with some patients also reporting numbness of the ipsilateral side of their face.

On examination of the ear there will be an extremely tender swelling in the external auditory canal, completely blocking it.

2.22.3 Management

Pope ear wick dressing with ciprofloxacin and hydrocortisone or dexamethasone for 48 hours will decrease the edema and should resolve the infection. A course of oral antibiotics and strong analgesia may be started if there are signs of severe disease, including significant edema and intense pain.

If the patient has diabetes, control of the disease is crucial. If patient is not known to have diabetes, but is experiencing recurrent boils in the ear, they should be screened for diabetes (using the HbA1C test).

The patient should be warned to avoid using Q-tips or hair pins for cleaning of their ear as they can cause injury to the outer canal, which can lead to infections and boil formation.

2.22.4 Essential facts

Any patient seen in primary care clinic with severe earache, to the extent that the ear cannot be examined, should be referred to an ENT clinic or the ED.

Chapter 3
Nose

3.1	Basic anatomy of the nose and sinuses	68
3.2	Differential diagnosis of nose problems	71
3.3	Rhinitis	72
3.4	Epistaxis	77
3.5	Sinusitis	80
3.6	Fracture of the nasal bone	83
3.7	Anosmia	85
3.8	Foreign body in the nose	88
3.9	Furuncle in the nose	89
3.10	Perforation of the nasal septum	90
3.11	Sleep apnea	92

3.1 Basic anatomy of the nose and sinuses

The nasal pyramid is made up of nasal bones, nasal cartilage, muscles, mucous membrane, and skin and together this unit forms an integral part of the face.

3.1.1 External nose

The external part of the nose begins from the root which lies between the eyes, the dorsum of the nose running down the middle, and its apex, which is considered the tip of the nose. The lower anterior part of the nose, called the nostril or anterior naris (singular; plural = nares), is built around a cartilaginous skeleton which is termed the upper and lower alar cartilage.

To some, the shape of their nose has significant esthetic implications; this needs to be recognized and addressed as appropriate.

3.1.2 Internal nose

The inside of the nose is divided by the nasal septum, which is made of bone in the upper part and cartilage in the lower part. The nasal cavity is lined with mucous membrane, except for the nasal vestibule which has a lining of skin. The cilia of the nasal lining move the overlying layer of mucus into the throat where it is swallowed. It then moves toward the stomach where acidic gastric contents can destroy any trapped substances. This mucus helps keep the nasal and sinus lining hygienic and free from irritants such as microorganisms, pollutants, and aeroallergens, e.g. dust.

The nasal cavity is surrounded by four walls (see *Figure 3.1*); its roof is formed by parts of the frontal, ethmoid, and sphenoid bones. The floor is formed by the palatine process of the maxilla and the horizontal plate of the palatine bone. The medial wall of the nasal cavity is formed by the nasal septum which is itself formed by the perpendicular plate of the ethmoid bone, the vomer, nasal crest of maxillary and palatine bone and cartilage. The lateral wall is prominent thanks to the three pillow-like processes which jut out – these are the superior, middle, and inferior turbinates, the space underneath which is termed concha (plural conchae). The nasolacrimal duct opens into the inferior nasal meatus, which is found below the inferior nasal concha. The nasal cavity opens posteriorly into the nasopharynx; this area is called the choanae.

The olfactory area lies over the superior one-third of the nasal cavity and here you will find the olfactory epithelium containing the olfactory neurons. These neurons join together to form the nerve bundles which run up through the cribriform plate of the ethmoid bone to the olfactory bulb in the brain. This olfactory tract transmits the sensory information to the olfactory center, which uses it to formulate the sense of smell.

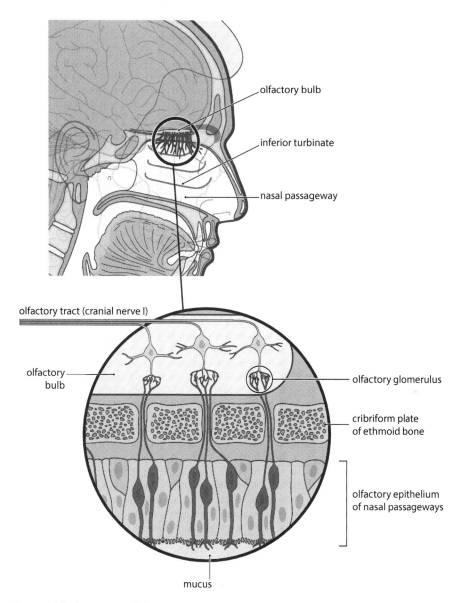

Figure 3.1 Basic anatomy of the nose.
Reproduced from *Anatomy and Physiology in Healthcare*, © Scion Publishing Ltd, 2017.

3.1.3 The paranasal sinuses

These are paired air-containing cavities in the maxillary, frontal, ethmoid, and sphenoid bones (see *Figure 3.2*). These sinuses are lined with mucous membrane and open into the nasal cavity. Their function is to lighten the skull and to give resonance to the voice; they are also responsible for producing mucus which protects the inner lining from pollutants, microorganisms, and aeroallergens such as dust.

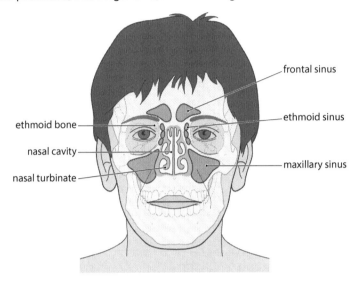

Figure 3.2 Basic sinus anatomy.

The maxillary sinuses are of a pyramidal shape and lie behind the cheek and over the roots of the premolar and molar teeth; they open into the nasal cavity via the *semilunar hiatus*. The frontal sinus is part of the frontal bone and is triangular in shape. It extends over the medial end of the eyebrow and backward to the orbit; this too opens into the semilunar hiatus. The sphenoid sinuses are found in the sphenoid bone and they open into *sphenoidal recesses* (these lie posterior and superior to the superior concha). The ethmoid sinuses are split into anterior, middle, and posterior and they are located in the ethmoid bone which is between the nose and eye. The anterior ethmoid sinus opens into the nasal cavity by the *infundibulum* (a passageway that opens into the semilunar hiatus groove in the ethmoid bone). The middle ethmoid sinus opens into the ethmoid bulla (this is a round swelling formed by the middle ethmoid cells and is found just above the semilunar hiatus) and the posterior ethmoid sinus opens into the superior nasal meatus which lies between the superior and middle conchae. Note that the *middle nasal meatus* is longer and deeper than the superior nasal meatus.

3.1.4 Vascular and nervous innervation

The nervous supply to the external nose is via branches of the trigeminal and ophthalmic nerves. As mentioned earlier, the sense of smell is via the olfactory nerve.

The external nose is supplied by branches of the maxillary and ophthalmic arteries, and the similarly named veins drain the nasal cavity. Lymph from the nasal cavity drains into submandibular and upper deep cervical lymph nodes.

3.2 Differential diagnosis of nose problems

The most common nasal concerns are listed below in the left-hand column, the differential for these concerns are listed in the middle column and the right-hand column shows in which section those conditions are described in more detail. The conditions are listed from most common to less common.

Symptom	Differential diagnosis	Section number
Congestion	Rhinitis	*Section 3.3*
	Deviated nasal septum	*Section 3.3*
	Sinusitis	*Section 3.5*
	Nasal polyposis	*Section 3.3.6*
Discharge from the nose (anterior and/or posterior)	Rhinitis	*Section 3.3*
	Sinusitis	*Section 3.5*
Epistaxis (see *Section 3.4*)	Fracture of the nasal bones	*Section 3.6*
	Perforation of the nasal septum	*Section 3.10*
Anosmia	Anosmia	*Section 3.7*
	Sinusitis	*Section 3.5*
Facial pain / pressure / headache / maxillary teeth pain / tenderness over the nose	Sinusitis	*Section 3.5*
	Fracture of the nasal bones	*Section 3.6*

Although you will be advised of specific investigations by the diagnosis in the relevant section (as above), the investigations detailed below are commonly used for nasal and sinus disease:

Tests in allergy / suspected allergy-mediated disease	Skin prick test Blood tests: RAST for specific allergens, immunoglobulin, ACE, ANCA *Aspergillus* precipitin test
Chronic disease or suspected mass lesion	Imaging with CT nose and sinus
Systemic disease or infection	CBC, ESR, CRP TFT and auto-antibody screen

3.3 Rhinitis

3.3.1 Introduction

Rhinitis is inflammation of the lining of the nasal passage. This can be for many reasons; see *Section 3.3.3*. It is common (incidence of up to 30% in the community) and is known to impact on quality of life, time away from the workplace in the relevant age groups, school achievement.

3.3.2 Diagnosis

A person suffering from nasal obstruction and/or sneezing and/or watery rhinorrhea and/or post-nasal discharge (usually mucoid) for at least an hour a day on most days is regarded as suffering from rhinitis. If there is associated sinusitis (see *Section 3.5*), the term *rhinosinusitis* is used; in this case there may additionally be headache and facial pain or pressure.

Patients may experience other symptoms too, including itching of the eyes or nose, diminished sense of smell and/or taste, or even associated hearing problems in some individuals.

Examination may reveal:
* *if co-existing sinusitis (whether this be acute or acute-on-chronic)* – there may be sinus tenderness
* *nasal lining* – appears hyperemic / blue / pale and boggy
* *nasal septum* – may be deviated or have a spur on it
* turbinate hypertrophy
* purulent drainage from the maxillary sinuses into nasal cavity
* nasal polyp (see *Section 1.2.2* for grading).

3.3.3 Causes

The table below shows the causes of rhinitis, grouped together.

Allergic	Seasonal
	Perennial
	Occupational
Non-allergic	Infective
	Non-infective

Allergic rhinitis

The triggers are usually airborne allergens. Seasonal allergic rhinitis is also colloquially referred to as 'hay fever' and is limited to certain months during the year (e.g. during pollen season). *Examples of common allergens*: grass, tree and weed pollen.

In contrast, perennial allergic rhinitis is where the allergen is present throughout the year, leading to year-round symptoms. *Examples of common allergens*: dust mite, cat, dog, mold and fungi.

In those with occupational rhinitis, their symptoms will resolve temporarily when away from the workplace and return when they go back to work. *Examples of common allergens*: flour, yeast, and latex.

Infective causes

- Viral (most common), bacterial, or fungal.

Non-infective causes

- Drug-induced
  - ○ e.g. aspirin, oral contraceptives, non-steroidal anti-inflammatory drugs (NSAIDs), antihypertensives (beta-blockers and hydralazine), alcohol (ethanol)
- Systemic diseases
  - ○ hypothyroidism, systemic lupus erythematosus, rheumatoid arthritis
  - ○ this form of rhinitis shows minimal/no response to conventional treatment
- Hormonal
  - ○ e.g. pregnancy
- Autonomic nervous system
  - ○ e.g. honeymoon rhinitis (can also be brought on by medication for erectile dysfunction)
- Congenital causes
  - ○ e.g. primary ciliary dyskinesia, cystic fibrosis
- Rhinitis medicamentosa
  - ○ this occurs secondary to medication overuse (in particular the inappropriate use of sympathomimetic decongestants which are used for nasal congestion)
- Idiopathic.

There is a phenomenon known as 'old man's drip', a condition whereby older patients suffer from watery rhinorrhea with no other symptoms or signs indicative of rhinitis and which shows minimal response to conventional treatment; this is *not* a form of rhinitis. For treatment, see the final paragraph of this section.

3.3.4 Investigations

There are three types of investigation exploring the cause of rhinitis, grouped below, to be requested as per your clinical diagnosis:

In allergy

- Skin prick test (preferable, but not covered by all insurances)
- Blood test: eosinophil count, RAST for specific allergens, total IgE count
- Nasal smear.

In systemic disease

- Blood test: CBC, CMP, ESR, TFTs, blood sugar level.

Immunology investigation

- Blood tests: ACE, ANCA, serum immunoglobulins, thyroid auto-antibody test
- *Aspergillus* precipitant.

Radiology

CT scan of the nose and sinuses should only be requested based on the severity or chronicity of the disease; for example, if despite a suggestive history and appropriate diagnosis the patient remains symptomatic on treatment or prior to possible surgery.

3.3.5 Management

Allergic rhinitis

Allergen avoidance advice is the treatment (nasal sprays, below, only address the problems developed due to allergen exposure).
- For example, in house dust mite allergy (causing perennial rhinitis) this includes anti-allergy bed mattress and pillow covers, no carpet or soft toys in the bedroom, and regular vacuuming and wet mop dusting of the room itself.
- In case of pet allergy, the pet should not be allowed in the bedroom and, if unable to part with the pet, no further pets should be acquired.

Intranasal steroid spray should be used regularly for a protracted period. It is crucially important that clear instructions are given on how to properly administer nasal sprays or nasal drops (see *Box 3.3.1*). Treatment failure is a very real (and unfortunately prevalent) consequence of inadequate treatment administration.
- This will target the inflamed nasal epithelium (secondary to exposure and reaction to allergen(s)).
- In case of pollen allergy (causing seasonal rhinitis) consider the use of a combination steroid and antihistamine nasal spray (instead of steroid only). It should be noted that insurances may not cover combination steroid and antihistamine nasal sprays, but often cover the two medications separately. Consider starting before the onset of the pollen season and discontinue once the season has finished.
- In severe cases, a short course of oral steroids may be indicated. Patients are frequently given a triamcinolone injection in primary care; this is often referred to as a 'snot shot'.

Antihistamine nasal sprays are especially helpful in those with itchy nose or bouts of sneezing. They need to be used more often but for a shorter duration, e.g. 3–4 times a day for up to 2 weeks, then reduce this to twice daily.

A *saline nasal wash* should be advised, preferably daily in the morning, during the pollen season.

In individuals whose allergic symptoms are not controlled and where symptoms are affecting quality of life consider *allergen-specific immunotherapy*.
- This may require referral to ENT or Allergy. Some primary care practices offer allergy immunotherapy.
- Immunotherapy is based on the results of allergy skin testing.
- Research has shown that in cases of seasonal and house dust mite allergy, desensitization for house dust mite first gives better results.

Non-allergic: infective

Acute viral infective rhinitis (experienced as the common cold) requires symptomatic treatment. Even in secondary bacterial infection (expect the duration of disease to be >1 week with purulent nasal discharge) studies have shown resolution of disease within 2 weeks without antibiotics; however, a benefit (albeit marginal) of using antibiotics after one week of disease has been noted.

Chronic infection may be more complex, especially if complications such as atrophic rhinitis (which can cause excessive crusting and a foul smell from the nose) require eradication of the underlying infection, as well as nasal wash to maintain nasal hygiene and steroid-based nasal drops to heal the epithelium.

Non-allergic: mechanical obstruction

Surgical correction is needed for abnormalities in the *nasal septum*, *turbinate* (e.g. surgical resection of enlarged inferior turbinate or submucus diathermy), or as treatment of *nasal polyposis*. Medical treatment for nasal polyposis can be considered first (see *Section 3.3.6*), before moving to surgical intranasal polypectomy or functional endoscopic sinus surgery with nasal polypectomy.

3.3.6 Essential facts

Nasal sprays can take up to 2 weeks to show their full benefit (when administered correctly and with good technique); patients should be counseled for this. Nasal sprays act locally and provided they are used within the recommended doses and limits, they should not cause considerable systemic side-effects.

Referral to ENT is indicated in a patient not responding to treatment (e.g. 6 weeks on the above treatment regime), if there are unilateral symptoms, nasal septal perforation, or the disease progresses, e.g. sinusitis or cellulitis (periorbital cellulitis needs urgent referral).

Nasal polyposis – medical treatment: this is based on steroid therapy; see example below:
- It is contraindicated in those for whom steroid therapy should be avoided or is associated with risk, e.g. tuberculosis (TB), blood pressure, peptic ulcer, glaucoma, diabetes, pregnancy, and psychosis.
  - Prednisolone 20 mg tid for 4 days and then decrease dosage for 14 days along with inhaled nasal steroid, most commonly fluticasone.
  - Review the patient in clinic with follow-up in 2 weeks.

Unilateral nasal polyp is an **ENT emergency** and should be referred to ENT as soon as the patient is seen in primary care clinic.
- In ENT the patient will undergo an endoscopic examination and CT scan of nose and sinus; if confirmed, they will need urgent nasal polypectomy with histology. In the case of antrochoanal polyps, patients should be observed every 6 months for the next few years as there is a 2% chance it will become malignant.

Patients are advised to do the saline nasal wash in the *morning* (see below). If they choose to do it in the late afternoon or evening, many patients report that the sinuses feel more congested that night, as the sinuses usually drain continuously for nearly half an hour after the wash. The correct ratio for saline rinse is 8 fl oz (250 ml) of water and 1 teaspoon (5 ml) of salt.

Excessive salt in the saline nasal wash will irritate the lining, leading to excessive mucus production by the epithelium. Consequently the maxillary sinus will fill up with this mucus and lead to even more nasal congestion, which is especially noted by patients at night.

In the case of *old man's drip*, ipratropium bromide nasal spray twice daily is the drug of choice (see *Box 3.3.1*). It should be given with caution to patients with prostatic hypertrophy and glaucoma.

Box 3.3.1 How to use a nasal spray / drops

How to hold the spray

- Hold it in your left hand when spraying into your right nostril and vice versa (see figure)
- Ensure that the nozzle of the spray, when in the nose, is pointing towards the outer wall of the nostril.
- Angle the nozzle slightly between sprays to ensure full coverage of the inner lining of the nose.

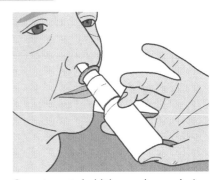

Correct way to hold the nasal spray device.

Method

1. Hold the spray and angle the nozzle as described above.
2. Take a breath in and hold it.
3. Push the spray bottle to administer the required number of doses.
4. Breathe out through the mouth.
5. Repeat if required.

Top tip

- For both the spray and drops, breathe gently after administering treatment; sniffing harshly will suck the treatment down into the throat.

How to use nasal drops

Hold the nasal drop bottle in the same manner as the nasal spray.

Correct positioning

Clinically, many patients favor the technique where they lie supine on the bed with a pillow under their shoulders, allowing their neck to be in an extended position.

Top tip

- Wait 1 minute after administering the nasal drops before moving, to ensure the medication has enough time to spread around the target area.

3.4 Epistaxis

3.4.1 Introduction

Epistaxis is bleeding from the nasal cavity; it can be unilateral or bilateral, into the anterior or posterior nasal space. It is a symptom rather than a disease and may sometimes require hospital admission. The peak ages of incidence are in children aged 2–10 and in adults aged 50–80 years.

3.4.2 Diagnosis

Most patients will notice epistaxis when it is coming from the anterior aspect of the nasal cavity; when it comes from the posterior aspect patients may also present with hemoptysis.

Examination is largely to confirm diagnosis and establish the bleeding site, not necessarily etiology. On examination, fresh blood or clotted blood may be visible in the nasal cavity. There may also be one or two dilated blood vessels stretching from the floor of the nasal cavity to the nasal vestibule. It is important to assess Kiesselbach's plexus (also known as Little's area); this is the most common origin site of epistaxis. It is located on the nasal septum bilaterally on the anterior aspect, and is a collection of blood vessels whose function is to provide nutrition to the septal cartilage. On examination of Little's area you may find dilated blood vessels and a bleeding site.

3.4.3 Causes

Most common	Accidental trauma / post-operative
	Anticoagulant therapy
	Secondary to high blood pressure
	Bleeding disorder
	Septal perforation
	Hemangioma / vascular polyp
	Acute infection of nose and/or sinuses
	Chronic nasal infections, e.g. granulomatosis with polyangiitis, atrophic rhinitis
Least common	Hereditary hemorrhagic telangiectasia
	Nasopharyngeal fibroma
	Malignant growth in the nose and/or sinuses
	Foreign body in the nose

3.4.4 Investigations

These should be selected according to the merit of the disease and clinical assessment of suspected cause.

Blood tests: CBC, CMP, international normalized ratio (INR), ESR, TFTs.

CT scan: nose and sinuses (rarely required).

Carotidangiography: in uncontrolled severe recurrent nosebleed.

3.4.5 Management

Home setting or primary care

Begin with conservative measures to halt the bleeding:
- Reassure the patient and ask them to maintain a seated position.
  - A nosebleed can be a very shocking and distressing experience, with some patients going into vasovagal shock because of it; keeping the patient safe and calm is of paramount importance.
- Instruct the patient to pinch the anterior portion of the nose using the thumb and index finger and hold for 10 minutes (patients frequently pinch only one side of the nose which can move the septum and thus decrease pressure). If there is still bleeding, spray into the nose 2 squirts of phenylephrine or oxymetazoline followed by pinching for 10 more minutes. If there is still bleeding then care in the ED is recommended.
  - Ask the patient to breathe through their mouth during this time.
- If available, an ice pack or pack of frozen food, e.g. peas, can be placed over the nasal bridge.
- Ensure the patient doesn't swallow the blood, as it may make them feel nauseated. If there is blood in the mouth, then simple cold water mouthwashes to rinse out the mouth should be adequate.
  - A bowl can be placed in front of the patient to spit out any blood in their mouth.

Hospital care

Care in this setting is aimed at directly controlling the bleeding by identifying and managing the bleeding site / cause.
- Prior to examination the clinician may place a cotton ball soaked with lidocaine and oxymetazoline in the anterior nares. This provides anesthesia and vasoconstriction, allowing better visualization and a degree of comfort for cauterization. If nasal examination identifies the bleeding site (e.g. a localized dilated vessel) then it can be cauterized using a silver nitrate stick after having gained valid informed consent from the patient.
- If it cannot be chemically cauterized (e.g. generalized profuse bleeding), the patient may require anterior nasal packing with ribbon gauze. Patients with nasal packing must be placed on antibiotics.
- In case of posterior nasal bleeding, posterior packing is required. These patients are generally medically frail and elderly and hospitalization is required.
  - Please note that there are many different types of products available in hospitals, which can be used according to the need.
- Some patients may benefit from a mild anxiolytic or sedative, as required.
- Surgical treatment may be required.

- A carotid ligation on the affected side may be recommended in uncontrolled or extreme cases.

In-hospital assessment needs to be carried out regarding consideration to temporarily withdraw any anticoagulant or antiplatelet medications.

Hospital care is also indicated to identify any signs of physical decompensation, through assessment and by recording and monitoring patients' vital signs.
- Depending on the volume of blood loss and patient factors, patients may require a blood transfusion.
- After recovery, patients may need a repeat check of hemoglobin levels or even a course of iron replacement.

Patients who have had posterior nasal packing will need to be observed for 24 hours once the packaging has been removed, before they can be sent home. Upon discharge the patient will still need to exercise caution, for at least 2 weeks. They should:
- avoid blowing their nose (especially in a forceful manner)
- cough and sneeze with an open mouth, and not pick their nose
- refrain from heavy or strenuous work
- when bathing (whether shower or bath), use only tepid water.

Patients are usually prescribed a topical nasal cream to apply twice a day for a week.

3.4.6 Complications

Depending upon the amount of blood loss and patient factors, the patient may go into hypovolemic shock (acutely) or become anemic (chronic). Therefore a thorough clinical assessment is required at the time, with appropriate follow-up thereafter.

3.4.7 Essential facts

- A considered and cautious approach, preferably by a hematologist, is needed for patients with known blood dyscrasia (e.g. hereditary hemorrhagic telangiectasia) or on medication increasing the tendency to bleed (e.g. anticoagulants or antiplatelet). This is particularly important because even minor trauma whilst treating the nose can lead to further extensive nosebleed.
- Patients with recurrent short bouts of epistaxis, which are usually amenable to conservative management, need referral to ENT to identify the underlying cause, investigate, and treat.
  - By obtaining CBC and coagulation profiles in advance, any abnormalities can be managed in primary care or the patient's coagulation clinic.

3.5 Sinusitis

3.5.1 Introduction

This is inflammation of the lining of air-containing hollow paired cavities in the skull, called sinuses. These sinuses open into the nasal cavity and are named the maxillary, ethmoid, frontal, and sphenoid sinuses.

3.5.2 Diagnosis

Patients may present with one or a constellation of the below symptoms:
- Nasal discharge
  - post-nasal or anteriorly
  - commonly yellow to green in color, although it can also be blood-stained
- Pain
  - facial pain and/or pressure; headache
  - toothache, usually worst first thing in the morning; pain increases with bending over
- Nasal obstruction
- Bad taste in the mouth
- Cough (see bottom of this list)
- A reduction in the sense of smell and taste
  - in severe cases, patient may complain of total anosmia or cacosmia
- Acid reflux/heartburn in those with acute-on-chronic rhinosinusitis
  - this is due to the post-nasal discharge (which comprises sub-clinically infective secretions which are swallowed) causing a related increase in acid production in the stomach to neutralize them
  - persistent symptoms lead to acid-induced irritation of the larynx; this in turn leads to cough and swelling of the interarytenoid region (leading to a foreign body sensation in the throat).

On examination: rigid nasal endoscopy

Nasal lining
- The nasal lining may appear blue to purple in color. It may look boggy/swollen, depending on the severity of the disease.
- A cobblestone appearance of the inferior turbinate may be noted in case of chronic infection in the nose and sinuses.

Nasal septum
- The lining of the nasal septum may also appear congested.
- Check for a deviated septum – this may impair drainage of the sinuses on that side.

Mucopurulent drainage or pus may be noted in the nasal cavity and post-nasal space. Pus may also be draining from the infected sinuses into the nasal cavity.

In cases of chronic infection, there will be excessive crusting in the nose.

Check for signs of previous nasal surgery; for example, maxillary antrostomy, open ethmoid air cells, or perforation of the nasal septum.

3.5.3 Causes

Most common	Infection (commonly viral or bacterial)
	Mechanical causes which affect the drainage of the sinuses / stasis of their secretions and infection, e.g. septal deflection, nasal polyp, nasal growth / malignancy
	Allergy-mediated
Least common	Secondary to mucociliary disorders, e.g. primary ciliary dyskinesia
	Dental infections leading to maxillary sinus through the root of tooth
	Sinonasal tumor (suspect if unilateral symptoms, facial swelling, or crusting)

3.5.4 Investigations

Blood tests: CBC, CMP, ESR.

Imaging: CT scan of nose and sinuses. Note that X-ray of paranasal sinuses is discouraged as CT scan is gold standard and provides the required information.

3.5.5 Management

Acute sinusitis

Begin with steam inhalation once daily for 3–5 minutes, or inhaled nasal saline.
- It works by moistening the air inside the lining, loosening the secretions and acting as a natural expectorant. It also helps relieve the spasm of surrounding muscles and ameliorates coughing and irritation of the throat.
- It works on the lining of nose and sinuses, throat, and upper chest.

Decongestant nasal spray / drops should not be used for more than 7–10 days at a time. Regular use can lead to rhinitis medicamentosa (inability to breathe without the vasoconstriction of decongestant sprays). Intranasal steroid spray has also been proven helpful, although its beneficial effects may take weeks to show.

In primary care antibiotics are not routinely recommended as most patients' disease resolves with the above measures (aimed at facilitating sinus drainage). It should be considered for those with severe symptoms, not improving / worsening symptoms over two weeks from onset. In resistant cases, immunomodulatory antibiotics are preferred for six weeks to three months, along with nasal wash and steroid nasal spray.

Chronic sinusitis

This is considered to be sinusitis lasting more than 6 weeks and etiology is more likely to be secondary to bacterial / fungal infection, allergy, or structural abnormalities (see *Section 3.5.3*). As such, treatment should be directed to the cause.

As with acute sinusitis, facilitating sinus discharge and treatment of infections with antimicrobial therapy is a mainstay. Intranasal steroids and allergen avoidance play a much greater role in allergy-mediated disease. Structural abnormalities will require specialist opinion and management. Prior to consideration of surgical treatment for chronic sinusitis, patients are generally treated with 'maximal medical therapy' by ENT.

Surgical treatment

For acute sinusitis not responding to medical treatment, an antral washout may be done under antibiotic cover; this can be performed under local or, where needed, general anesthetic. This procedure is rarely performed in the US.

Other surgical procedures for recurrent chronic sinusitis (depending upon the severity and chronicity) might include intranasal antrostomy, Caldwell–Luc operation (rarely), and, more commonly, functional endoscopic sinus surgery. In case of frontal sinusitis not responding to treatment, individual surgical intervention is needed.

3.5.6 Complications

These are not very common but can be serious and include orbital cellulitis (review for eye symptoms, visual acuity or pain on eye movement), osteomyelitis of the surrounding bones, meningitis, abscesses (e.g. extradural, sub-dural, or intracranial).

3.5.7 Essential facts

Immunocompromised patients are at a much greater risk of aggressive fungal or bacterial infection.

In 80% of cases it is the maxillary sinus which is involved first; if untreated, other sinuses are involved and this is called pansinusitis.

Sinus infection is not isolated – it always co-exists with rhinitis or nasal inflammation and frequently allergic rhinitis.

Only a small proportion of patients managed with the above treatment regime in primary care do not respond, or suffer recurrence. If the patient is getting recurrent sinus infections (≥3 per year), they need a course of antibiotic and if they remain symptomatic between episodes (sinus pain / pressure or excessive post-nasal discharge) consider referral to otolaryngology for evaluation of chronic sinusitis. Cases of suspected complication development would need an immediate referral.

3.6 Fracture of the nasal bone

3.6.1 Introduction

This is discontinuity of the nasal bones, with or without displacement, in the nasal pyramid.

3.6.2 Diagnosis

Patients may present with history of facial trauma, epistaxis, external nasal swelling, external nasal deformity, nasal obstruction, and/or decrease or loss of sense of smell.

On examination, depending on the severity of the fracture (e.g. displaced nasal bones vs. a greenstick fracture) the associated swelling will be proportional (e.g. a greenstick fracture may have soft tissue swelling only). It is important to note that the associated swelling of the nasal pyramid can last up to 4 weeks after nasal trauma.

Check for a septal hematoma, which is seen as a bilateral nasal septal swelling. It can lead to septal abscess which looks like a nasal septal swelling with a paler tinge; this can cause complete nasal obstruction.

3.6.3 Causes

Of all the causes of fracture, by far the most common is accidental trauma to the nose bones. These should be assessed by emergency care / ENT specialists.

3.6.4 Investigations

In simple uncomplicated fractures, no investigations are required. In serious injuries, motor vehicle accidents, or cases of intentional trauma / physical abuse cases, X-rays have a strong medicolegal value.

Imaging: a CT scan of nose and sinuses is advised, depending upon the severity and complexity of the fracture.

3.6.5 Management

When there is external nasal deformity with no soft tissue swelling, the fractured nasal bone requires surgical intervention in the form of manipulation and reduction of the fractured nasal bone under anesthetic. This should be done within 2 weeks of the injury otherwise more radical surgery, in the form of rhinoplasty or septorhinoplasty, may be required.

Where there is an open wound, the patient should be treated with a course of oral antibiotics, local dressings of the wound, and regular follow-up until the wound has healed.

If there is a septal hematoma or abscess, urgent incision and drainage is needed, otherwise it could lead to nasal disfigurement.

3.6.6 Complications

The external nasal deformity can have a significant impact on a patient's psychology.

The deviated nasal septum can impair drainage of the sinuses, leading to nasal and sinus disease.

The nasal septal cartilage gets its blood supply from the overlying mucous membrane. In case of trauma to the mucosal lining or separation of the lining from the septum (due to a septal hematoma or abscess), this deprives the cartilage of its nutrition. This leads to necrosis of the septal cartilage, which causes sagging of the nasal bridge. This is seen clinically as a saddle-shaped nose.

3.6.7 Essential facts

- If the patient develops nasal and sinus symptoms after nasal trauma, they should be referred to otolaryngology.
- A fracture of the ethmoid labyrinth or a skull fracture involving the cribriform plate can cause a discharge of CSF (presenting as clear nasal discharge). This can be tested for by performing a beta transferrin test on the liquid. If the test is positive, the patient needs an emergency neurosurgical referral for further management.

3.7 Anosmia

3.7.1 Introduction

This condition is characterized by the inability to recognize common smells in the normal environment. A reduced sense of smell is called hyposmia. Some patients also complain of an associated loss of sense of taste.

3.7.2 Diagnosis

This is a subjective symptom and is not easy to quantify clinically in primary care / basic setting (more extensive tests are carried out in specialist centers). Often a good screening question is whether patients are able to identify the smell of smoke / burning (e.g. burning toast) in their home. Remember that a detailed history needs to be carried out, investigating allergies, systemic disease, trauma, and acute or acute-on-chronic nasal and sinus infections. Also take a medication history and family history.

On examination of the ENT (see *Section 1.2*), check for mechanical obstruction (e.g. deviation of the nasal septum or a nasal polyp) or signs of infection (pus in the nasal cavity or pus draining from the sinus(es) into the nasal cavity).

It is always important to perform a neurological and systemic examination when assessing for anosmia / hyposmia.

3.7.3 Causes

Most common	Rhinitis (viral)
	Rhinosinusitis (acute / chronic)
	Nasal polyposis
	Septal deviation
	Post-operative
	Nasal growth
	Hypothyroidism
	Epilepsy
	Drugs
Least common	Neurological conditions: • e.g. tumors (meningioma of the olfactory groove, ethmoid tumors, frontal lobe, multiple myeloma), head injury involving cribriform plate • e.g. infection – meningitis • e.g. neurodegenerative disease – Kallmann syndrome
	Idiopathic

3.7.4 Investigations

Investigations will help to establish the underlying cause.

Allergy: skin prick test, RAST for specific allergens.

Infection or systemic disease: blood tests including CBC, CMP, TFTs and thyroid auto-antibodies, ESR, ACE level and ANCA.

Mass lesion: imaging using CT scan of nose and sinuses, involving olfactory pathway.

3.7.5 Management

Symptom-specific advice

Intranasal steroids, on a long-term basis, may be required to address any underlying swelling causing blockage of aromas through the nasal pathway. Targeted locally absorbed sprays usually have very minimal systemic effects. In some cases, a short course of oral prednisolone may be needed in severe or refractory acute-on-chronic disease.

For symptomatic relief, a trial of zinc supplements can be initiated for 2 months; some find it helpful (this should not delay investigation for a serious underlying pathology). The theory behind this is that the olfactory cell contains zinc granules and, theoretically, a deficiency of these granules can lead to anosmia.

Treating the cause

Note that the patient with a history of anosmia or hyposmia should be referred to ENT sooner rather than later for further assessment, investigation, and treatment of said cause, due to the severe nature of some of the causes (see above).

See *Sections 3.3* and *3.5* for details of treatment of the nasal or sinus infection, respectively.

Surgical correction of any mechanical obstruction (e.g. septal deviation, nasal polyp, or nasal growth) should be planned where indicated – refer to otolaryngology for surgical consideration.

3.7.6 Essential facts

A small group of patients, 10–15%, who develop anosmia due to a severe cold, flu or acute rhinosinusitis, will improve with the passage of time; however, complete recovery is not guaranteed.
- The theory behind the improvement in sense of smell in these cases is that there is a reduction in the swelling of the lining of the nose, sinuses, and around the olfactory area which was formerly impairing the passage of aromas to the olfactory area for detection and interpretation.

- Those whose sense of smell does not recover when the swelling decreases have suffered damage to the cilia and mucosal nasal lining and function of the nasal olfactory lining, leading to long-term or permanent damage to the sense of smell.

Anosmia can be a sign of neurological (including some neurodegenerative) diseases; hence referral to ENT and possibly Neurology for investigation, diagnosis, and treatment should be completed.

Safety around the home

- It is imperative that patients have working fire alarms around their home, especially in high risk areas such as the kitchen.
- It is important to check and clearly highlight the expiration date on food to ensure spoilt food is not ingested by mistake.

3.8 Foreign body in the nose

3.8.1 Introduction

Patients are usually young children (up to 2 years old) brought to ENT emergency or outpatient clinics with either a history of or an incidental finding of a foreign body in the nose.

3.8.2 Diagnosis

In small children, there is usually a history of unilateral foul-smelling nasal discharge. In older children, where there may be history of previous events, the foreign body is usually obvious on examination of the nose, even by just raising the tip of nose.

3.8.3 Causes

Common foreign bodies include beads, stones, pieces of building block, popcorn, tissue paper, or pieces of jewelry.

3.8.4 Management

Specialists should extract the foreign body on their *first* attempt upon examining the patient.

In non-/minimally cooperative or very young children extraction should be done under short general anesthesia. The airway should be protected in case the foreign body enters the nasopharynx or larynx, which would cause further complications including airway compromise.

3.8.5 Essential facts

At primary care level, removal of a foreign body should not be attempted. Children may not be optimally cooperative (whether out of fear or pain) and specialist instruments are required; hence the patient should be seen in ENT emergency clinic.

3.9 Furuncle in the nose

3.9.1 Introduction

This is an infection of the hair follicles in the nasal vestibule and is commonly caused by *Staphylococcus aureus* infection.

3.9.2 Diagnosis

Patients will complain of severe pain, swelling and tenderness at the tip of the nose along with generalized symptoms of fever, malaise, and/or myalgia.

Furuncles can be seen in either of the nasal vestibular areas of the nose. On examination, the infection site appears inflamed, being hot, red, and tender to touch. Note that anterior rhinoscopy for examination is very painful for the patient.

3.9.3 Causes

Furuncles in the nose are commonly due to a bacterial infection by *Staphylococcus aureus*. One of the risk factors for developing this is those who are in the habit of picking their nose, thereby causing digital trauma and introducing infection into the hair follicle.

3.9.4 Management

When a patient is seen in primary care clinic and the furuncle appears fluctuant, the patient should be referred to ENT for incision and drainage along with antibiotics and analgesia. If the abscess is more indurated then oral antibiotics and analgesics with follow-up within 3 days will suffice.

3.9.5 Complications

A serious complication is cavernous sinus thrombosis (suspected if there is swelling of the upper lip, pain in eye / head with worsening symptomatology). This requires emergency referral to ED as admission is required for intravenous antibiotics, observation, and further management.

3.9.6 Essential facts

A screening test for diabetes should be considered on a first presentation, but especially in recurrent cases. Diabetes mellitus, especially when there is poor control or a new diagnosis, can predispose to infections; a boil in the nose is one of the infections which may present.

Be sure to educate patients for signs of cavernous sinus thrombosis and advise them to seek immediate attention if such signs develop.

3.10 Perforation of the nasal septum

3.10.1 Introduction

This is a hole in the nasal septum.

3.10.2 Diagnosis

This normally presents with non-specific symptoms such as epistaxis, blocked nose, nasal bridge pain or tenderness over the nose. One of the few specific symptoms is when patients complain of a whistling sound from their nose, related to their breathing.

Examination is to confirm the site of the perforation, granulation tissue, excessive crusting in the nose or the presence of fresh to clotted blood.

3.10.3 Causes

Most common / Least common	
Surgery on the nose
Trauma to the nose
Idiopathic
Recreational drug use, e.g. inhalation of cocaine and, more recently, opiates
Granulomatosis disease of the nose

3.10.4 Investigations

Investigations mainly comprise blood tests to look for systemic disease (e.g. autoimmune conditions) or infection. Tests include CBC, CMP, ESR, CRP, ACE level, ANCA and syphilis serology.

3.10.5 Management

Medical

Medical management is use of a nasal wash and application of Vaseline in the nasal cavity. If infection is present, treat with the appropriate antimicrobial topical antibiotic nasal cream in the recommended dose. In some cases oral therapy may also be required.

Surgical

Surgical treatment is via insertion of a prosthesis. However, in the long term there is a risk that the prosthesis may fall out or cause recurrent nasal infection which can, in some cases, lead to an increase in size of the perforation.

3.10.6 Complications

Chronic nasal crusting and chronic nosebleed can lead to recurrent nasal and sinus infection and anemia.

3.10.7 Essential facts

At primary care level, whenever there is suspicion of septal perforation the patient should be referred to ENT for investigation and treatment.

3.11 Sleep apnea

3.11.1 Introduction

This is defined as cessation of breathing during sleep for at least 10 seconds at a time. Usually termed 'obstructive sleep apnea' (OSA), as opposed to central sleep apnea, it is caused by anatomical narrowing or poor muscle tone in the upper airway or oropharynx.

3.11.2 Diagnosis

During the night it may be noted that the patient snores loudly. The patient may be tired, feel they lack a good night's sleep, or experience daytime somnolence. They may also suffer from morning headaches, have symptoms associated with chronic hypoxia and be chronic mouth breathers. Children may display behavioral problems, particularly in school.

Sleep apnea can also have a wider impact, causing poor work performance, forgetfulness, anxiety, depression, and even enuresis.

On examination look out for signs causing the pathology: nasal polyp, gross deflection of nasal septum, turbinate hypertrophy, or nasal growth. Be sure to inspect the throat and overhanging uvula and soft palate.

3.11.3 Investigations

Polysomnography (sleep study) is the standard method of diagnosing and evaluating sleep apnea.
- It includes an EEG, ECG, eye movement monitoring, monitoring of respiratory rate and oxygen saturations. Additional monitoring of the nasal and oral airflow, and movement of the legs or arms and chin is carried out.
- The number of apneic episodes is recorded. More than 5–10 per hour in the context of the history and examination is highly suggestive of sleep apnea. Oxyhemoglobin desaturation is also noted and is another index which can be used for diagnosis; if it is <85% it too is highly suggestive of sleep apnea.
- Respiratory disturbance index, also called apnea / hypoapnea index, is the total number of apnea to hypoapnea episodes per hour of sleep. Fewer than 5 episodes is regarded as normal. Up to 30 indicates a mild apnea, and 30–50 with oxygen saturation less than 85% would be classed as moderate disease. Severe sleep apnea is when the score is 50 and oxygen saturation 60%.

The Epworth Sleepiness Scale questionnaire evaluates the subjective symptoms of disrupted sleep. Clinically obstructive sleep apnea is diagnosed if the Epworth score is >12 and BMI is >30. However, sleep apnea is now frequently seen in non-obese patients.

Other tests are requested based on the merit of the disease and suspected underlying cause and include chest X-ray, CBC, and TFTs.

3.11.4 Management

Conservative management consists of weight loss (if patient is overweight) with dietitian advice where possible.

If an underlying infection is suspected, treat as per *Sections 3.3* and *3.5*. If systemic disease is suspected, e.g. hypothyroidism, review the relevant guidelines and pathways.

The remaining interventions will need specialist input.

Mechanical devices

These include continuous positive airway pressure (CPAP) ventilation via nasal or oral mask to maintain airway patency. This is regarded as being highly effective; however, some machines are known to make a significant amount of noise when in use.

Tongue and mandibular positioning devices have been successful in reducing snoring apneic events and improving oxygen saturation.

Surgery

Uvulopalatopharyngoplasty is the most common surgical procedure for obstructive sleep apnea in the US. This procedure includes tonsillectomy, trimming of the posterior edge of the soft palate and uvula. Laser-assisted uvuloplasty is also an option. This surgical intervention for snoring has a record of only limited success in the long term.

In the case of gross deviation of the nasal septum, a septoplasty is indicated. If nasal polyposis or sinus infection are involved, then functional endoscopic sinus surgery with nasal polypectomy is recommended.

3.11.5 Complications

Untreated patients can have increased workload on their heart and develop cardiac complications in the long term.

3.11.6 Essential facts

Patients with loud snoring, with or without <u>witnessed</u> sleep apnea, should be referred to ENT for investigation and treatment.

Chapter 4
Throat

4.1	Basic anatomy of the throat	96
4.2	Differential diagnosis of throat problems	98
4.3	Dysphagia	100
4.4	Tonsillitis	103
4.5	Peritonsillar abscess	106
4.6	Pharyngitis	107
4.7	A change in voice	109
4.8	Laryngitis	112
4.9	Stridor	114
4.10	Acute epiglottitis	118
4.11	Aphthous ulcer	120
4.12	Salivary gland stones	121
4.13	Foreign body in the throat	123
4.14	Halitosis	124
4.15	Neck mass	126

4.1 Basic anatomy of the throat

The throat contains numerous active organs, connections, muscles, nerves, and lymphatics within it (see *Figure 4.1*). Those directly involved in ENT are explained below; however, the reader is reminded to keep an open mind when assessing the throat and esophagus and its pathology.

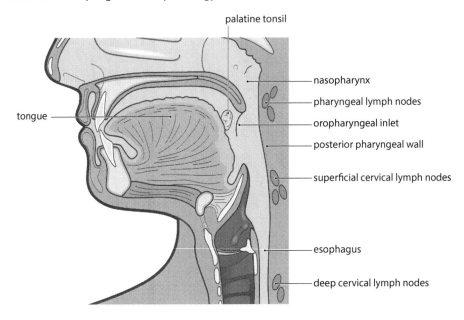

palatine tonsil

nasopharynx

pharyngeal lymph nodes

tongue

oropharyngeal inlet

posterior pharyngeal wall

superficial cervical lymph nodes

esophagus

deep cervical lymph nodes

Figure 4.1 Basic anatomy of the throat.

4.1.1 Gastrointestinal / esophageal tract

The primary function of the gastrointestinal (GI) tract is ingestion of foodstuffs and digestion to absorb nutrients and excretion. The oral cavity begins the process when it receives food and uses mechanical (chewing) and chemical (salivary enzymes, glands as below) destruction to make a food bolus which is then swallowed. The largest and most commonly recognized salivary glands are the parotid (whose oral opening is found in the mouth, opposite the 2nd maxillary molars), submandibular (the opening of which is in the floor of the mouth under the tongue), and sublingual (which open near the frenulum of the tongue) glands.

The tongue is of great importance in this process, both in terms of mechanical breakdown of food and taste sensation. The sensation of taste is supplied by the chorda tympani branch of the seventh cranial nerve (the facial nerve), which supplies this to the anterior two-thirds of the tongue. The sensory nerve supply of the oral cavity is through branches of the fifth cranial nerve (the trigeminal nerve). Blood supply and drainage of the oral cavity are through branches of carotid vessels.

The throat contains two major connecting tubes, one of which is the esophagus, which is a muscular tube 18–25 cm in length. It connects the oral cavity to the stomach.

The oropharyngeal inlet is formed anteriorly by the base of the tongue and the lingual tonsils, the palatine tonsils on the sides and posteriorly (superior aspect) by the nasopharynx and the posterior pharyngeal wall. This collection of lymphoid tissue forms a ring at the oral inlet along with the superficial and deep cervical lymph nodes of the neck; they are all involved in the local immune response to oral pathogens.

4.1.2 Respiratory tract / airway

The primary function of this system is to allow for gaseous exchange of oxygen into the blood circulation and removal of carbon dioxide from the blood. See *Section 3.1* for further details on the anatomy of the nose. Starting from the nasopharynx (see *Figure 4.1*), its connection to the lower respiratory tract is via the trachea (the second of the major connecting tubes found in the throat).

Around the level of the hyoid bone lies the hypopharynx which consists of the epiglottis (a flap-like structure protecting the trachea from aspiration; see *Figure 4.2*), paired aryepiglottic folds, and arytenoid cartilages, commonly known as the laryngeal inlet.

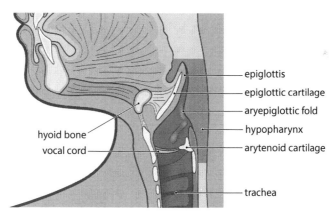

epiglottis
epiglottic cartilage
aryepiglottic fold
hypopharynx
arytenoid cartilage

hyoid bone
vocal cord

trachea

Figure 4.2 Basic anatomy of the epiglottis.

The larynx extends from the epiglottis to the cricoid cartilage and includes the vocal folds. The larynx contains multiple cartilages and muscles that serve in voice production. Beyond this is the trachea and then lung tissue, i.e. the lower respiratory tract.

4.1.3 Functional roles: speech

The lips, tongue, teeth, and secretions from mucous glands found in the oral cavity, all play integral roles in the articulation of speech.

4.2 Differential diagnosis of throat problems

Perform a clinical assessment of the patient, as shown in *Sections 1.1* and *1.2*. In the left-hand column of the table below are the most common presenting symptoms of throat disease, and the center column shows the differential diagnoses, in order of prevalence in terms of causative pathology for the index symptom.

Symptom	Differential diagnosis	Section number
Dysphagia	Acute infections of throat, nose, larynx, and pharynx	*Sections 4.6, 3.3, 4.8*
	Gastroesophageal reflux disease (GERD)	
	Foreign body in the throat	*Section 4.13*
	Esophageal stricture – benign or malignant	
	Achalasia cardia	
	Corrosive burns	
	Pharyngeal pouch	*Section 4.3*
	Goiter	
	Globus pharyngeus	
	Multiple sclerosis	
Odynophagia	Acute infections of larynx, pharynx, and tonsils	*Sections 4.6, 4.8, 4.4*
	Peritonsillar abscess	*Section 4.5*
	Trauma due to foreign body in the throat	*Section 4.13*
Sore throat	Viral infections of the upper respiratory system, e.g. tonsillitis (rarely bacterial)	*Section 4.4*
	Peritonsillar abscess	*Section 4.5*
	Acute infections of throat, nose, larynx, and pharynx	*Sections 4.6, 3.3, 4.8*
	Glandular fever (also known as mononucleosis, or just "mono")	*Section 4.4*
	Chemical irritation, e.g. pollutants, allergy, smoking (latter two causing chronic sore throat)	–
	Gastroesophageal reflux disease (GERD)	
Change in voice	Acute infections of throat, nose, larynx, and pharynx	*Sections 4.6, 3.3, 4.8*
	Overuse / traumatic	
	Local mass lesions	
	Malignancy of upper lung or other tissue around the recurrent laryngeal nerve (causes vocal cord palsy)	*Section 4.7*
	Iatrogenic, e.g. recent thyroid or parathyroid surgery	
	Secondary to inhaled corticosteroid use	
	Systemic disease, e.g. thyroid disease, allergy-mediated reaction	

Symptom	Differential diagnosis	Section number
Stridor	Infection	*Section 4.10*
	Anaphylactic reaction	*Section 4.9*
	Foreign body in the throat / larynx	
	Trauma	
	Other: hereditary angioneurotic edema, stenosis at any level, laryngomalacia, tumors	
Oral pain	Aphthous ulcer	*Section 4.11*
	Salivary gland stone, infection, and tumors	*Section 4.12*
	Foreign body in the throat	*Section 4.13*
Halitosis	Acute infections of throat, nose, and pharynx	*Sections 4.6, 3.3, 4.8*
	Dental infection / poor dental hygiene	*Section 4.14*
	Aphthous ulcer	*Section 4.11*
	Antibiotic use	*Section 4.14*
	Endocrine abnormalities: ketosis, fasting, alcohol	
	Systemic disease	
Trismus	Peritonsillar abscess	*Section 4.5*
	Salivary gland stone, infection, and tumors	*Section 4.12*
	Dental pathology	–
Neck mass	Acute infections of throat, nose, larynx, and pharynx	*Sections 4.6, 3.3, 4.8*
	Mononucleosis	*Section 4.4*
	Salivary gland infections, stone, and tumors	*Section 4.12*
	Thyroglossal cyst	*Section 4.15*
	Branchial cyst	
	Lymphoma	
	Metastatic carcinoma from post-nasal space, pharynx, larynx, lungs and abdomen, breast, and thyroid	

4.3 Dysphagia

4.3.1 Introduction

Dysphagia is a difficulty or abnormality in swallowing, ranging from a minor discomfort to complete obstruction. It has huge implications for the patient's oral intake and risk of dehydration. The history of presenting complaint is very helpful in focusing the encounter, especially to establish onset and whether it is associated with pain.

4.3.2 Diagnosis

Odynophagia is not a specific symptom but is more likely to indicate a throat pathology (see *Figure 4.3*) or corrosive burns (if the history is indicative of this). Throat and laryngeal pathologies can also cause referred pain to the ear, causing **otalgia**.

A change in or hoarseness of voice, **dysphonia**, may indicate laryngeal pathology; infection will cause congestion of the larynx, acid reflux will cause interarytenoid edema which impairs vocal cord function. Mass lesions such as malignancy of vocal cords will cause nodules, leading to a physical impairment of the vocal cords.

The **sensation of a lump** in the throat, noted **swelling** or a pressure sensation over the **anterior neck** need to be explored thoroughly as these could be due to acid reflux, enlarged thyroid of any cause or a malignancy (especially if relevant risk factors are found in the history). A systemic review of thyroid symptoms and identification of any unexplained **weight loss** should be considered.

Esophageal or upper GI pathology may be indicated if the patient complains of associated **dyspepsia**, a **metallic taste** in the mouth, or **regurgitation** of food in the mouth. Such pathologies may also cause a **cough** as the acidic secretions irritate the larynx; however, respiratory pathology should be excluded in a patient with a cough.

4.3.3 Causes

The causes of dysphagia can be split into the four categories shown in the table below.

Most common ↓ **Least common**	Throat	Infection
		Foreign body
	Esophagus	GERD
		Benign stricture
		Achalasia cardia
	Structural	Goiter
		Pharyngeal pouch
		Malignancy, anywhere in the pharynx, larynx, or upper GI tract
	Functional	Multiple sclerosis
		Globus pharyngeus

The associated symptoms and past medical history will aid in narrowing the differential diagnosis, with examination greatly assisting the establishment of a diagnosis.

Throat examination

Look for ulcers or any dental pathology:
- Inspect the oral cavity carefully, including tongue and posterior pharyngeal wall.

Inspect the tongue for white coating (may be brown in a smoker), which may indicate fungal infection.

Assess the palatine tonsils:
- Look at their size, any asymmetry or presence of prominent crypts
- Look for cheesy white material in the tonsillar crypts (tonsilloliths).

Assess the lingual tonsils for size and asymmetry.

Flexible nasopharyngoscopy

This is usually done by an ENT specialist and is crucial to assess the lower pharynx and larynx. Nasopharyngoscopy allows for examination of:
- Base of the tongue
- Lingual tonsils
- Epiglottis / vallecula
- True and false cords
- Arytenoid and interarytenoid regions (note if there is any edema)
- Piriform fossa (look for the presence of cysts or growths).

Neck examination

Examine the neck, as shown in *Section 1.2.3*.

Assess for any swellings and be sure to relate these to the swallow motion. If a swelling is noted, palpate it and define it, as shown in *Section 1.2.3*.

Check for any lymphadenopathy.

4.3.4 Investigations

These are requested upon the merit of the disease and your working diagnosis.

Blood tests: CBC, ESR, TFTs, iron profile.

Imaging: Barium swallow with or without video fluoroscopy, chest X-ray, ultrasound scan (USS) of the neck, panendoscopy with biopsy and histology if suspected lesion is visualized.

4.3.5 Management

This is dependent on the cause; see *Section 4.2* for further details. As a general concept, infections are usually managed with conservative management and, if needed, antibiotics or antifungals.

A structural abnormality, e.g. pharyngeal pouch, will need surgical review for potential excision. Should malignancy be suspected, the patient must be urgently referred to Otolaryngology for biopsy, staging, and treatment planning (which may include surgical excision, chemotherapy, or radiotherapy). It is important to remember the high risk these patients have of having an obstructed airway; hence specialist input is key in advance planning for this.

Patients with dyspepsia (also known as acid reflux) should be reviewed for **ALARM Symptoms** (**A**nemia – iron deficiency, **L**oss of weight, **A**norexia, **R**ecent onset of progressive symptoms, **M**elena / hematemesis, **S**wallowing difficulty / dysphagia) and signs indicating that they may need further investigation for serious pathology. Dyspepsia should be treated with advice on diet and eating habits and, if required, pharmacotherapy of antacids +/− proton pump inhibitors (PPIs).

Achalasia is a neuromuscular disorder preventing free passage of food from the esophagus to the stomach, leading to gross dilatation of the distal esophagus above the lesion. Medical treatment with drugs to reduce the lower esophageal sphincter, such as calcium channel blockers or long-acting nitrates, is limited. Botulinum toxin injection can be helpful along with dilatation of the esophagus. Laparascopic myotomy (a procedure whereby the lower esophageal sphincter has an incision made in it) with partial fundoplication is generally the most recommended surgical procedure.

A pharyngeal pouch is when the pharyngeal mucosa between the upper and lower parts of the inferior constrictor muscle (thyropharyngeus and cricopharyngeus) herniates through the dehiscence of Killian in the midline, posteriorly. Treatment is surgical, ranging from simple dilatation of the stricture to endoscopic division of the wall between the pouch and the esophagus by diathermy or Dohlman's procedure. A large pouch will need excision of the pouch.

Globus pharyngeus should only be diagnosed when GERD or peptic ulcer disease has been excluded (many may even require upper GI tract endoscopy). It is a condition where reassurance of the absence of malignant or serious causative condition needs to be given and for the patient's fears and concerns to be explored and addressed. This may require specialist input.

4.3.6 Essential facts

Post-cricoid carcinoma usually affects middle-aged women with chronic iron deficiency anemia. This is usually referred to as Plummer–Vinson syndrome, or sideropenic dysphagia, and is the development of an esophageal web associated with iron deficiency, presenting with dysphagia. On examination clinical signs include koilonychia, glossitis, and angular stomatitis. It is a pre-malignant condition requiring specialist review.

4.4 Tonsillitis

4.4.1 Introduction

The palatine tonsils are a collection of lymphoid tissue located at the back of the oral cavity laterally (see *Figure 4.3*). Acute infection is most common in the 5–15 year age group. Tonsillar infection usually involves surrounding tissue, to an extent, leading also to a recognized pharyngitis.

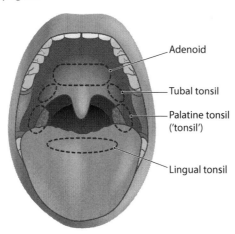

Adenoid

Tubal tonsil

Palatine tonsil
('tonsil')

Lingual tonsil

Figure 4.3 Tonsils in the oral cavity.

4.4.2 Diagnosis

The most specific symptom of tonsillitis is sore throat; other symptoms may include foul breath and malaise, with or without pyrexia. Examination may reveal tonsillar enlargement, with or without pus visualized over the tonsils, prominent tonsillar crypts, and cervical lymphadenopathy (in particular the jugulodigastric lymph nodes).

The associated pharyngitis may be indicated by pain or difficulty swallowing and, on examination, an inflamed oropharynx may be visualized.

Examination findings consistent with chronic tonsillitis would include anterior faucial flare and cheesy material seen on the tonsillar crypts (though the latter may also occur in acute infection) and persistently palpable jugulodigastric lymph nodes (which drain the tonsils).

4.4.3 Causes

Infection is the commonest cause, usually viral in nature. When bacterial (approximately 15–30% of cases), the most common causative bacteria is Group A beta-hemolytic *Streptococcus*. Predisposing factors include malnourishment and overcrowded living conditions.

An exceedingly rare cause, but with important clinical implications, is tonsillar tuberculosis. The affected patient should be screened for TB risk factors. Tonsillar malignancy should be excluded in the case of unilateral tonsillar enlargement.

4.4.4 Investigations

These should be requested depending upon the merit of the disease and if additional tests are required to exclude other differentials.

Laboratory tests: rapid strep., throat culture, heterophile antibodies (monospot), CBC.

4.4.5 Management

Simple analgesia should be offered, along with conservative management options with rest and staying well hydrated. Most cases are self-limiting; however, **Centor criteria** have been developed to identify those patients who are most likely to have a sore throat secondary to Group A beta-hemolytic *Streptococcus* and may benefit from antibiotics:

- Tonsillar exudate
- Tender anterior cervical lymph nodes
- Absence of cough
- History of fever.

Having three or more of these signs suggests the incidence rate of 40–60% for said bacterial infection and such patients may benefit from antibiotics. The antibiotic of choice is usually penicillin (or azithromycin/erythromycin if penicillin-allergic); however, practices vary.

Care should be taken to avoid the use of ampicillin and amoxicillin, which may precipitate an acute rash if the patient has mononucleosis.

4.4.6 Complications

In general, these are uncommon. The development of a peritonsillar abscess (see *Section 4.5*) has an incidence of 2% in cases of severe acute tonsillitis. Other complications include infection of surrounding structures (ear – OM; sinus – acute sinusitis; neck – abscess). However, antibiotic use has been shown to reduce the risk of all these.

Thanks to the greater use of antibiotics, the incidence of rheumatic fever (autoimmune complications of acute streptococcal tonsillitis) is exceedingly rare in developed countries. However, in developing countries it is still a significant cause of morbidity and, rarely, mortality.

4.4.7 Essential facts

When to refer for tonsillectomy: the criteria

A history of recurrent acute tonsillitis (requiring antibiotics) 3–4 times a year during which a patient requires time off work/school, for at least two consecutive years, would allow the patient to be considered for tonsillectomy. Only rarely will insurance companies approve tonsillectomy with less frequent occurrences.

Other causes of tonsillectomy are if uvulopalatopharyngoplasty (a surgical procedure for OSA; see *Section 3.11*) is being undertaken or there is a suspected neoplasm in the tonsil. The size of the tonsils themselves is not a criterion for tonsillectomy unless they are causing obstructive symptoms or there is asymmetry in tonsillar size.

Frequently tonsillectomy is indicated in children, even if tonsils are healthy, if they are enlarged and causing obstruction in breathing or sleep apnea. This can easily be determined in a sleep lab with a sleep study.

Tonsilloliths

These are a collection of cheesy material in the tonsillar crypts. They cause significant distress for many patients who have typically already tried removal with water picks and hydrogen peroxide gargles. But they are asymptomatic and in most cases do not need any treatment other than mouthwash, maintaining good hydration and eating foods with hard surfaces, e.g. pear, apple and meat, along with some vegetables.

Some patients keep assessing their throat in the mirror and try to remove these tonsilloliths using Q-tips or even their fingernails, which can lead to infection and bleeding and should be completely avoided. Tonsillectomies are frequently approved by insurance companies for tonsilloliths and are commonly performed.

4.5 Peritonsillar abscess

4.5.1 Introduction

Peritonsillar abscess, once commonly referred to as quinsy, is the development of a pus-filled collection outside the tonsillar capsule (usually communicating with the tonsil at the upper pole).

4.5.2 Diagnosis

There is usually a history of acute tonsillitis (it is a known complication of this; see *Section 4.4*) which is not improving, the presence of trismus (reduced opening of the jaw), otalgia (referred pain phenomenon), vocal changes, and severe dysphagia (objectively seen as drooling of saliva out of the mouth).

On examination, the most indicative finding is unilateral swelling in the peritonsillar space. This, and the subsequent edema, causes deviation of the uvula. Also notable on physical examination is the audible classic 'hot potato' voice.

4.5.3 Management

If the patient has inadequate oral intake and is at risk of dehydration, they should be admitted for intravenous antibiotics and fluids until oral intake of fluids is tolerated.

The patient needs emergency ENT review for assessment and potential management. A peritonsillar abscess requires incision and drainage using local anesthetic and antibiotic. Referring the patient to ED may facilitate obtaining an emergency CT and admission.

These patients also need to be considered for tonsillectomy as soon as possible after the initial episode, which is usually after 6 weeks, although in some it may be later. It is important, as patients may suffer from recurrences without it and have worse symptoms, with impact on quality of life in the later flares.

4.6 Pharyngitis

4.6.1 Introduction

The pharynx is a hollow tubular space (see *Figure 4.4*). It is exposed to pathogens via the inhaled and ingested route and at risk of indirect infection via spread from infected surrounding structures.

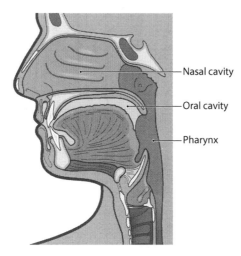

Nasal cavity

Oral cavity

Pharynx

Figure 4.4 Anatomy of the pharynx.

4.6.2 Diagnosis

This condition lacks specific symptoms or signs. It is usually associated with tonsillitis or nasal infections, leading to an overlap at presentation with these symptoms (sore throat with dysphagia, or nasal congestion, respectively). Examination will reveal an erythematous pharyngeal mucosa and relevant findings associated with any concurrent infection.

4.6.3 Causes

Infections are usually viral in origin. Apart from adenovirus and common influenza infection, important viral pathogens to be aware of are rhinovirus, measles, mononucleosis, and typhoid fever. Bacterial pharyngitis is less common; however, if present the most common pathogen is Group A *Streptococcus*, or diphtheria which is more prevalent in developing countries. Also be aware that common pathogens causing STIs (*Neisseria gonorrhoeae, Chlamydia trachomatis*, and *Treponema pallidum*) may infect the throat.

It is important to be aware that some important immunodeficient states may present with pharyngitis as the presenting symptom; these include:
- agranulocytosis
- leukemia
- HIV infection.

4.6.4 Investigations

These should be requested based upon the merits of the disease. Common investigations include the following.

Rapid strep test and rapid antigen detection test.

Throat culture: send to the lab to isolate the pathogen (especially important to do if you suspect bacterial infection).

Blood tests: CBC, CRP, and ESR (infection markers), renal function (assessing for renal impairment as a consequence of dehydration), and CMP.

4.6.5 Management

This should include liquid diet, bed rest and appropriate analgesia. If you suspect bacterial infection, penicillin is recommended and should be started unless the patient is allergic.

It is advised to avoid ampicillin and amoxicillin in glandular fever as these may cause a rash to develop.

4.6.6 Complications

Although rare, bacterial infection can lead to abscess development in peritonsillar or parapharyngeal spaces. In those cases secondary to Group A beta-hemolytic *Streptococcus*, thanks to the greater use of antibiotics, the incidence of rheumatic fever (autoimmune complications of acute streptococcal infection which may include cardiac complications) is exceedingly rare in developed countries. However, in developing countries it is still a significant cause of morbidity and mortality.

4.6.7 Essential facts

Of clinical interest is the fact that syphilis can cause a generalized pharyngitis and on examination there will be highly infective snail track ulcers.

Chronic pharyngitis is usually due to non-infective causes such as smoking, excessive alcohol intake, or mouth breathing (which could be secondary to chronic rhinosinusitis), which should be treated according to the cause.

In case of chronic pharyngitis, hypertrophy of posterior pharyngeal lymphoid tissues contributes to the symptoms, which may require cryotherapy or cautery under general anesthetic.

4.7 A change in voice

4.7.1 Introduction

This is a change in the normal tone and pitch of the voice resulting in either a hoarse, weak, croaky, or husky voice. Some patients may suffer from aphonia for a period of a few hours to several days.

4.7.2 Diagnosis

The history of presenting complaint may be difficult to explore extensively if the patient is finding it difficult to speak and is not accompanied by someone who can help with the history; it is important to establish onset, pain (may be referred pain in the ear, in case of laryngeal or dental pathology), and checking for associated symptoms of infection and trauma (as above). Risk factors should be ascertained for malignancy and the patient's past history needs to be reviewed for iatrogenic causes.

Begin with a general examination, identifying signs of infection (erythema of the back of the throat, enlarged tonsils +/– exudate) or thyroid disease. Laryngeal examination, especially in secondary care where direct visualization by endoscopy is available, is helpful. The findings and their implications are as follows:
- Generalized congestion of larynx → infection, acid reflux
- Vocal cord polyp / papillomatosis / neoplasia → as indicated
- Vocal cord paralysis → nerve palsy, aortic aneurysm, malignancy of larynx
- Closure of false cord earlier than true cords → voice abuse, acid reflux
- On palpation, tension at the region of larynx → voice abuse, vocal cord polyp or nodule.

4.7.3 Causes

Most common ↓ **Least common**	Infection	Affecting larynx, throat, or sinuses *(viral or bacterial)*
	Overuse / trauma	Excessive singing / shouting
		Coughing / vomiting
		Direct neck trauma
		Inhalation of noxious fumes
	Mass lesions	Polyps – idiopathic / singer's nodule
		Papilloma
		Malignancy of the larynx
		Malignancy of upper lung or other tissue around the recurrent laryngeal nerve *(causes vocal cord palsy)*
	Iatrogenic	After intubation
		Post thyroidectomy / parathyroidectomy
		Post radiotherapy
		Secondary to inhaled corticosteroid use *(causes myopathic weakness of muscles of the vocal cords)*
	Systemic	Thyroid disease
		Allergy-mediated reaction

4.7.4 Investigations

These are dependent upon your working diagnosis and the merit of the disease.

Blood tests: CBC, CMP, ESR, and TFTs.

Imaging: Chest X-ray, videostroboscopy, CT scan of chest involving recurrent laryngeal nerve pathway.

4.7.5 Management

Lifestyle changes which will support the larynx include smoking cessation and limiting actions which are considered vocal abuse, e.g. coughing, shouting, and excessive singing, especially without prior vocal training exercises. Consider referral to speech pathology for patients who are subject to vocal cord overuse occupationally. If the patient has known allergies, appropriate avoidance measures are key and the patient should take extra care to maintain good hydration levels.

Speech therapists can provide a valuable service to support patients in specific cases including head and neck cancer patients. ENT specialist referrals depend on the working diagnosis; infections and some overuse / trauma causes may be managed in primary care, with referral considered if inadequate improvement in 2 weeks. Where mass lesions or iatrogenic causes are being considered, prompt referrals are recommended.

Specific management should be advised according to diagnosis and merit of the disease. Patients with dyspepsia (also known as acid reflux) should be reviewed for **ALARM S**ymptoms (**A**nemia – iron deficiency, **L**oss of weight, **A**norexia, **R**ecent onset of progressive symptoms, **M**elena / hematemesis, **S**wallowing difficulty / dysphagia) and signs indicating that they may need further investigation for serious pathology. The dyspepsia should be treated with advice on diet and eating habits and, if required, pharmacotherapy of antacids +/– PPIs.

Infections are usually treated conservatively (see *Section 4.6*) unless there are complications or bacterial infection is suspected.

Should thyroid disease be identified, it is important the patient is stabilized, and reviewed by endocrinologists.

Mass lesions (e.g. vocal cord polyp / growth; see *Section 4.7.3*) will require surgical excision by an otolaryngologist.

4.8 Laryngitis

4.8.1 Introduction

The larynx (colloquially known as the voice box) is found inferior to the pharynx (see *Figure 4.5*). Although it is small there are many key structures here and it is important to remember that any of these can be involved. Its function is to produce sounds and protect the trachea from aspiration.

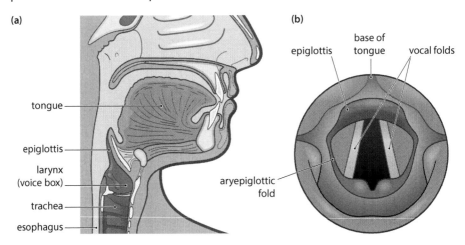

Figure 4.5 Anatomy of the larynx.

4.8.2 Diagnosis

The distinctive symptom in laryngitis is an intermittent change in the voice (which is usually secondary to inflammation of the vocal cords); the remainder of the symptoms are non-specific. Red flag signs for malignancy include progressive worsening in voice with stridor, dysphagia, otalgia, and a neck mass on examination.

Outside of obvious vocal quality, examination is normally unremarkable for specific signs for laryngitis, but is key in order to identify associated pathology such as tonsillitis and rhinosinusitis. Although it is difficult to differentiate viral from bacterial laryngitis clinically, fungal infection may be indicated by white spots on the base of the tongue with diffuse laryngeal edema.

4.8.3 Causes

Infection is the most common cause of acute laryngitis; other causes include irritant exposure (e.g. smoking or excess ingestion of alcohol), allergens, trauma (e.g. overusing the voice, excessive coughing), and malignancy.

Note that laryngitis secondary to infection is usually associated with infection of the surrounding tissues, e.g. pharyngitis or upper respiratory tract infection. Bacterial and viral infection can co-exist, i.e. initial viral infection with opportunistic superimposed bacterial (where patients will get acutely worse over time).

Fungal infection accounts for approximately 10% of these cases. Risk factors for the development of this include recent use of antibiotics, diabetes mellitus, and use of inhaled corticosteroids.

4.8.4 Management

Acute laryngitis secondary to infection is usually self-limiting (lasting less than 2 weeks), although if it is suspected to be bacterial in origin or the patient is systemically ill with fever or purulent drainage, they may require antibiotics.

Lifestyle measures including resting the voice (until the patient no longer has any pain or discomfort, range 3–7 days). Be sure to advise patients to refrain from whispering, as this strains the voice more than conversational speech. Other specific advice includes reducing caffeine intake, staying well hydrated, and avoiding sitting in air-conditioned areas; such measures will aid recovery.

Educate the patient to seek emergency care immediately if airway compromise is suspected or impending (see *Section 4.9*). This is especially important in young children.

4.9 Stridor

4.9.1 Introduction

This is high pitched, noisy breathing due to airflow obstruction because of airway narrowing. It is an emergency because there may be imminent airway compromise (though there are some stable chronic causes, see below) if it is not managed appropriately.

4.9.2 Diagnosis

It is important to ascertain whether or not the stridor is acute; if so, the common causes seen clinically are *foreign body* (indicative history or **very acute onset** of symptoms, i.e. from seconds to minutes) or *infection* (**fever**, **odynophagia**, **contact**); these should therefore be excluded immediately. Though rare, *anaphylaxis* too has a very sudden onset; however, there is usually a trigger (commonly bee sting or food allergens) and history of allergy. An airway assessment to identify if *respiratory compromise* is imminent should be performed immediately; see below.

The characteristics of the stridor are helpful in identifying the potential site of the lesion (see *Figure 4.6*). When stridor is predominantly inspiratory, the suspect obstruction is thought to be above (or at) the vocal cords; alternatively, when predominantly expiratory it is likely to be below this (i.e. bronchial). Associated symptoms are helpful in further localizing this: when inspiratory and associated with **snoring** this is more likely to indicate nasal pathology; however, when inspiratory but associated with some **dysphonia** it may point to a pharyngeal or laryngeal pathology. Stridor which is equally inspiratory and expiratory is likely to be tracheal.

Signs of acute respiratory distress

Check to see if the patient appears distressed and clinically unwell. Also check for cyanosis, pallor, tachypnea, low oxygen saturation, flaring of the nares, use of accessory respiratory muscles for breathing (subcostal/intercostal recession – a see-saw movement of the abdomen with breathing), tracheal tug, poor air entry, and/or added sounds such as wheeze on auscultation.

Throat

Assess for signs of an acute infection which may be present including fever, erythema of the posterior throat, gross enlargement of the tonsils with or without exudate, and lymphadenopathy.

Larynx

Refer to ENT for nasopharyngoscopy. The key findings that should be assessed for are generalized congestion in the larynx, any growth seen in the larynx or foreign body noted.

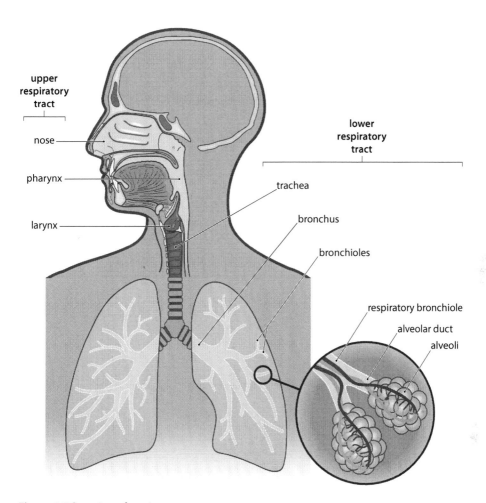

Figure 4.6 Overview of respiratory tract anatomy.

4.9.3 Causes

Most common ↕ **Least common**	Infection	Acute laryngitis
		Acute epiglottitis
		Acute laryngotracheobronchitis (croup)
		Bacterial trachiitis
		Diphtheria
	Structural	Anaphylactic reaction
		Foreign body in the throat
		Hereditary angioneurotic edema
		Stenosis at any level (chronic), e.g. cysts, vascular rings
		Congenital laryngomalacia
		Tumors: laryngeal, lung
	Traumatic	Direct trauma to the neck
		Inhalation of toxins (leading to edema)
		Post-intubation

4.9.4 Investigations

These are largely to investigate for infections; see *Sections 4.8* and *4.10*.

Specialist imaging can be used for structural causes; however, this is usually requested by specialists and is dependent on the merit of the disease.

4.9.5 Management

If you suspect acute respiratory compromise or imminent emergence of this, then the patient needs urgent and prompt review by specialists (primarily in ED) so that the airway can be safely managed. Ensure that the patient doesn't become distressed as this can only worsen the situation.

Foreign bodies are visualized and treated via laryngoscopy by ENT / anesthetics in the operating room. Severely ill patients need assessment for tracheostomy.

See *Sections 4.8* (laryngitis) and *4.10* for specific management of infections. Please note that although exceedingly rare, diphtheria (with its classical pseudomembrane over the tonsils / soft palate and oropharynx), is an important cause of stridor, especially in the unimmunized community. When in hospital it is managed by antidiphtheria toxin (although there is a small risk of anaphylaxis with this) and the unimmunized are given vaccination.

Patients with stridor caused by trauma should be reviewed by ENT urgently.

If a neoplasm is suspected or visualized on examination a referral to otolaryngology is required to exclude malignancy via biopsy, determine staging, and treatment planning which should be discussed with the patient and family.

Hereditary angioneurotic edema is due to a deficiency in C1 inhibitor; the airway needs close monitoring as there is a risk of compromise. Acutely it is treated with C1 inhibitors; however, tracheostomy can also be considered if there is progressive disease. Patients should be seen at least once annually by a specialist in the condition.

Structural congenital conditions such as stenosis, usually beginning in childhood, need to be reviewed by specialists; the patient/caretaker will be able to discuss the management of either watchful waiting or surgery with the specialist.

Laryngomalacia causes intermittent stridor, usually triggered by an acute upper respiratory tract infection when the child cries or is sleeping. It accounts for approximately two-thirds of all congenital stridor. ENT review, particularly by a pediatric otolaryngologist, recommended for assessment and regular follow-up of these children, where required.

4.10 Acute epiglottitis

This is an ENT emergency, as it can be fatal.

4.10.1 Introduction

The epiglottis becomes infected, leading to localized edema of the epiglottis and supraglottic larynx. Classically it affects those aged 2–6 years; however, the *H. influenzae* immunization has decreased the occurrence in this age group. In the last 25 years, cases are more commonly seen in adults, but keep in mind that children sometimes do not receive recommended immunizations.

4.10.2 Diagnosis

The symptoms include dysphagia with high grade temperature which rapidly develops into a change in voice and respiratory obstruction (which may even be more pronounced than the stridor).

Clinically the child appears unwell; scared, drooling, and quiet. They frequently sit in the "tripod" position. It is imperative that you **DO NOT examine the patient's throat** as this may precipitate acute obstruction.

4.10.3 Causes

Haemophilus influenzae type B is the most common cause; however, a vaccination is available for this (see above).

4.10.4 Investigations

This is a clinical diagnosis; it is advised to do nothing that will upset the patient – this includes doing blood tests and anything that may cause anxiety (e.g. taking child away from parents). There needs to be prompt management of the airway and thus no delays, such as above.

Imaging

- Performed in the operating room with an anesthesiologist present, the patient will undergo rigid laryngoscopy for direct visualization of the epiglottis and airway management.
- A lateral neck X-ray is requested only when the airway is secure or the specialists are present, if immediate intervention is needed. A markedly enlarged epiglottis, classically called the 'thumbprint sign', is seen on film.

Blood tests

- Do not need to be performed immediately if patient is in distress.
- CBC, CMP, infection markers – CRP.

Microbiology

- Blood cultures
- Throat culture – ONLY when airway secured by specialist.

4.10.5 Management

The airway needs to be secured immediately. If seen in primary care, recommend / arrange immediate ambulance transportation to the ED.

Once the airway is maintained and intravenous antibiotics are given, patients improve quickly; however, they require close monitoring until resolution. Steroids, antipyretics, and analgesics are also recommended as the combination of drugs will treat the patient effectively and quickly.

4.10.6 Complications

Acute air obstruction.

Less commonly: infection of surrounding tissue – neck, mediastinum, lung (pneumonia).

4.10.7 Essential facts

In adults the condition is usually slower in onset but they also have a slower recovery. Adults have a lower intubation rate (approximately 20%) compared to that in children, the majority of whom require this.

Acute laryngotracheobronchitis (or croup) is a viral infection which affects the subglottic region (cf. supraglottic epiglottitis). Affected children are usually less than 2 years old and have a barking cough, inspiratory stridor, thick secretion, low grade fever, and minimal, if any, dysphagia. There may be repeat episodes. Treatment is with humidified air and, if not improved, steroids. If the patient remains symptomatic pediatric referral is important. It should not be taken lightly as severe croup may necessitate patients being intubated and ventilated or surgical intervention in the form of a tracheostomy.
- Hospitalization should be considered for anyone whom you suspect as suffering from epiglottitis, i.e. showing respiratory distress, abnormal clinical parameters (e.g. hypoxic, cyanotic) or who appears clinically ill (pallor).

Bacterial tracheitis is similar to acute epiglottitis; it affects children usually, with dysphagia, stridor, and a clinically sick or toxic-looking child. **It is an emergency**, to be dealt with in hospital, and great emphasis is placed on keeping the situation calm and giving antibiotics which are the drugs of choice.

4.11 Aphthous ulcer

4.11.1 Introduction

Aphthous ulcers are shallow, painful lesions on the mucosal surface of the inner mouth and along the tongue.

4.11.2 Diagnosis

The primary symptom is that of localized pain; however, depending on location they can also cause severe pain in the throat.

Examination usually reveals a well-circumscribed lesion with a central pallor and surrounding erythema. Be sure to check for other lesions in the mouth also, and any surrounding lymphadenopathy.

4.11.3 Causes

The cause can be local trauma; for instance, dental trauma can cause ulcers on the tongue due to constant irritation. It is sometimes related to systemic disease, such as Behçet's, celiac or Crohn's. Sometimes it is related to stress or it can even be idiopathic.

4.11.4 Investigations

If the ulcer has not resolved within 2 weeks it is advisable to refer for a biopsy to exclude a malignant lesion.

The following are requested in cases of recurrent ulcers, to identify any systemic disease:

Blood tests: CBC (anemia), iron profile + B_{12} + folate (hematinic screen), total immunoglobulin A and IgA tissue transglutaminase (celiac screen).

4.11.5 Management

Most will resolve on their own without scarring. Those not resolved within 2 weeks need investigation to exclude malignancy (as above) and ENT referral.

Symptomatic relief can be achieved through topical application of a soothing analgesic, e.g. benzydamine hydrochloride, or 'Magic Mouthwash'. In recurrent ulcerations, dexamethasone ointment has been shown to be helpful.

If the ulcer is due to local irritation, then resolving the index cause (e.g. rectifying any dental deformity) plus local treatment of the ulcer, will heal it.

4.12 Salivary gland stones

4.12.1 Introduction

There are two paired salivary glands: the parotid gland and submandibular gland. Other glands include the submental glands and many mucous sublingual glands. If calcified stones deposit in the outflow tracts of these glands they can obstruct them, causing pain and increasing the risk of infection. Stones usually occur in adults and are rare in children.

4.12.2 Diagnosis

The patient may present with pain, swelling, and infections, possibly recurrent, of the affected gland. On examination of the oral cavity there may be swelling and tenderness on bimanual palpation of the gland. The stone may actually be visible in the duct opening, particularly Wharton's duct.

In cases of submandibular gland stone (the most common location of all salivary gland stones, accounting for up to 90% of all), this painful swelling is related to eating, especially in the acute phase. As well as trismus (difficulty in opening the mouth) patients may have symptoms consistent with infection, including fever and generalized malaise.

4.12.3 Causes

The cause of stone development is unclear; however, it is thought that the submandibular gland is most affected due to its anatomy and its secretions being more viscid. It is also thought that oral bacteria and the salinity of saliva result in the formation of calcification / stones.

4.12.4 Investigations

This is dependent upon the merits of the disease.

Blood tests: CBC, ESR.

Imaging: US of the neck and affected gland with FNA, sialogram (to explore the salivary gland and its tract), or CT scan of neck (when assessing for a mass in the salivary gland).

4.12.5 Management

In case of acute infection, broad-spectrum antibiotics are recommended.

For recurrent flares, an ENT referral is recommended; if the stone is in an opportune location, it can be removed from the submandibular duct through minor surgery in an ENT outpatient clinic, which can be a source of great relief for the patient. In the majority of the cases, if symptoms are recurrent, treatment is excision of the affected gland with histopathology of the sample.

4.12.6 Essential facts

Children with suspected stones should be referred to otolaryngology.

Stones in the submandibular gland are usually singular and large; those in the parotid are smaller and multiple.

A ranula is a swelling in the floor of the mouth, secondary to rupture of the salivary gland and it comprises retained mucus – patients need to be evaluated by an ENT specialist.

Salivary gland tumors make up approximately 7% of all head and neck cancers. As with stones, they present with pain, but on examination there is usually a hard and fixed lump, sometimes causing overlying skin ulceration. The majority are in the parotid gland; in fact approximately 70% of parotid swellings are benign pleomorphic adenomas and the remainder are cysts or lymph nodes. Tumors in the smaller salivary glands in the mouth are more likely to be malignant. In any case these require urgent referral to be assessed, investigated, and managed by specialists.

4.13 Foreign body in the throat

4.13.1 Introduction

The most common foreign bodies to become lodged in the throat are fish bones, pieces of chicken bone or meat in adults. In children the usual age group is 3 years and older, as children start exploring coins and other small items and, through curiosity, put them into their mouth.

4.13.2 Diagnosis

Symptoms include the sensation of something being stuck in the throat, odynophagia, dysphagia, drooling of saliva, and even vomiting. In case of a fish bone, patients may give a history of a foreign body being stuck for a period of a few hours through days or even weeks.

On examination, fish bones are often seen to stick to the lower pole of the tonsils. They can be removed with forceps, providing instant relief to the patient. It is advisable that this is done in the ED or an otolaryngology clinic.

4.13.3 Management

Patients with history of foreign body ingestion should be referred to the ED.

If no foreign body is seen, sometimes a scratch or injury to the pharynx or tonsillar mucosa may be the source of the symptoms. On occasion the base of the tongue may show some localized inflammation, and there may be a scratch or swelling. In these cases, X-ray of the neck (lateral view) is important to exclude the foreign body.

Usually no active treatment is required apart from simple analgesia for a few days.

In the case where no foreign body is visualized and simple analgesia is required, the patient should be reassured that there is no foreign body and that there shouldn't be any further complication. Despite this, if symptoms persist, very rarely, the patient may need to be examined under general anesthetic via endoscopy.

4.14 Halitosis

4.14.1 Introduction

This subjective problem sometimes presents itself to ENT clinic.

4.14.2 Causes

Infection	Tonsillitis, pharyngitis
	Nasal and sinus infections
	Bronchiectasis
	Chest infection
Oral cavity	Dental infection / poor dental hygiene
	Ulcerative lesions such as aphthous ulcers
	Antibiotics *(may alter normal oral and pharyngeal flora)*
Endocrine	Fasting
	Ketosis
	Alcohol
Other	GERD
	Sjögren syndrome
	Renal failure

There are a wide range of varying causes for true halitosis. A good history, with a robust systems review, and thorough clinical examination will help to support or refute the diagnosis.

Focusing on the ENT examination, look in the throat for any ulcers and dental / tonsillar / pharyngeal infection. The visualization of the larynx may show congestion or interarytenoid edema. Examining the nose may reveal congested nasal lining and infective secretions (yellow–green in color).

4.14.3 Investigations

These will be based upon the working diagnosis and may include the following:

Blood tests: CBC, ESR, CMP (includes U&E and LFTs), blood glucose reading.

Microscopy: throat culture.

Imaging: chest X-ray.

4.14.4 Management

This includes improving oral hygiene, adequate hydration, treating the cause and reassurance (where appropriate).

It is recognized that this symptom is difficult to treat in primary care clinic if there are no specific history or examination findings, hence patients are usually referred to an ENT specialist or dentist.

4.15 Neck mass

4.15.1 Introduction

The neck is anatomically split into the anterior and posterior triangle (see *Figure 4.7*). Location is key to determining what the potential diagnoses are.

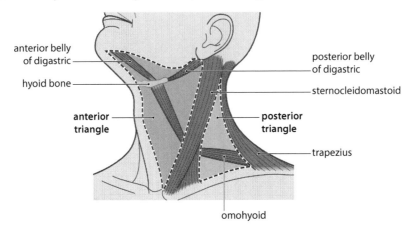

anterior belly of digastric

hyoid bone

anterior triangle

posterior belly of digastric

sternocleidomastoid

posterior triangle

trapezius

omohyoid

Figure 4.7 Anatomical triangles of the neck and their borders.

4.15.2 Diagnosis

The patient may note the lump subjectively and may be suffering from consequences of this (dysphagia, sensation of lump in the throat, pain; see *Section 4.15.3*) or the associated symptoms of the underlying condition (malignancy or hypo- / hyperthyroidism).

Patients should be examined as outlined in *Section 1.2.3*. Note that one of the most common midline neck swellings is a thyroglossal duct cyst. An enlargement of the left supraclavicular lymph node (known as Virchow's node) is often associated with intra-abdominal malignancy such as colon or stomach cancer.

4.15.3 Causes

The list of causes can be extensive and is based upon the underlying anatomy. Some of the most common causes seen clinically are:
- acute infections of throat, nose, larynx, and pharynx
- glandular fever
- thyroid goiter / nodule
- salivary gland infections, stones, and tumors
- thyroglossal cyst
- branchial cyst

- lymphoma
- metastatic carcinoma from post-nasal space, pharynx, larynx, lungs and abdomen, breast, and thyroid.

4.15.4 Investigations

These are determined by your working diagnosis and the significance of the disease.

Blood tests: CBC, ESR and CRP (infection/inflammation markers), TFT +/– thyroid auto-antibodies and autoimmune screen (if lesion is suspected to be thyroid in origin).

Imaging: US of the neck (*Section 1.7.2*), sialogram (*Section 1.7.3*), chest X-ray, CT of the neck.

4.15.5 Management

This depends on your working diagnosis; see *Sections 3.3*, *4.6* and *4.8* for the management of acute infection. Endocrinology referrals are indicated for benign thyroid masses and an ENT referral should be considered for salivary gland disorders or a suspected thyroglossal cyst, to allow for further radiological investigations and FNA, or surgical removal, as required. If malignancy is suspected, the history should be used to identify the probable primary cause and referral is to that particular specialty (i.e. head and neck or upper GI).

Chapter 5
Pediatric ENT

5.1	Introduction	130
5.2	Guide to ENT issues covered elsewhere	131
5.3	Pediatric history taking	132
5.4	Rhinitis	135
5.5	Sinusitis	136
5.6	Epistaxis	138
5.7	Nasal trauma	140
5.8	Obstructive sleep apnea	141
5.9	Adenoiditis	143
5.10	Cystic fibrosis	144
5.11	Hearing loss and deafness	145
5.12	Acute otitis media	147
5.13	Tinnitus	149
5.14	Vertigo	150
5.15	Laryngeal papillomatosis	152

5.1 Introduction

Pediatrics is the healthcare service dedicated to those under the age of 18. As such, it covers life at a time when the mind and body are changing and developing rapidly. Understandably each stage varies in its healthcare needs. *Table 5.1* shows the recognized subdivisions of age to help address children's particular needs (may vary slightly between sources).

Table 5.1 Subdivisions of age in pediatrics

0–1 months	Neonate
1 month – 2 years	Infant
2–6 years	Young child
6–12 years	Child
12–18 years	Adolescent / young person

Upper respiratory tract symptoms and infections, with associated spread to the ear, are common in children. Often fleeting, they can in some cases cause significant impairment of hearing and quality of life and can even impact on academic achievement. There are a few acute airway-related ENT emergencies not to be missed in this age group.

This part of the book will take you through common and serious ENT diagnoses and their management.

5.2 Guide to ENT issues covered elsewhere

Much information is given within the sections of this chapter regarding the specifics of ENT problems as they relate to children. However, readers should be aware that much more detail is given in the original section covering a particular complaint. The right-hand column of the table below shows in which section complaints are more generally covered.

Ear	
Decreased hearing, hearing loss	*Section 2.3*
Foreign body in the ear	*Section 2.2*
Otitis media	*Section 2.7*
Tinnitus	*Section 2.18*
Vertigo	*Section 2.15*
Nose	
Epistaxis	*Section 3.4*
Foreign body in the nose	*Section 3.8*
Obstructive sleep apnea	*Section 3.11*
Rhinitis	*Section 3.3*
Sinusitis	*Section 3.5*
Throat	
Acute epiglottitis	*Section 4.10*
Foreign body in the throat	*Section 4.13*
Tonsillitis	*Section 4.4*

5.3 Pediatric history taking

5.3.1 General pediatric history

Most children do not usually present with complex histories or multiple co-morbidities. Commonly, there is a particular symptom of concern to the parents or patient for which they want treatment and reassurance that it isn't 'serious'. The information that can be gained from a good 'collateral' (from someone close to the child, e.g. a parent / guardian), is of great value in a pediatric history, where it is available.

A pediatric history is a narrative of the patient's current ill health in the context of several particulars about their growth and development. These are acknowledged through the addition of the following subheadings to the standard history (as seen in *Section 1.1*):

- General health review
  - ○ oral intake (feeding)
  - ○ sleep habits
  - ○ history of allergies
  - ○ immunizations
- Birth history
  - ○ antenatal, delivery and post-partum history
  - ○ to be asked in clinically relevant cases – unlikely to be needed in a young person's history
- Developmental history
  - ○ achievement of key milestones
  - ○ height / weight
  - ○ in clinically relevant cases
- Detailed social history
  - ○ who lives at home, any smokers at home, pets, any concerns at school?

Here is a concise acronym that can be used to support you to remember the key aspects of a general pediatric history: **GABDeS** → **G**eneral history including **A**llergies, **B**irth history, **De**velopment history, detailed **S**ocial history. Different sources may have variations on subheading names and distribution of content; however, the key themes remain consistent.

5.3.2 Introduction to an ENT history in pediatrics

Impairment of the ENT system can lead to reduced quality of life, poor growth, and inadequate development of the special senses, if not addressed promptly and properly.

Anatomically, children have a relatively larger tongue compared to their oral cavity, and thus their airway is more likely to become obstructed than an adult's. Infants (see *Table 5.1* for distinction) breathe exclusively via their nose and will experience respiratory distress if their nose is blocked – a clinically common phenomenon usually secondary to infection. Infections of the nose can easily travel up to the ear via the

Eustachian tube (see *Figure 2.1*), as it is horizontal (as opposed to diagonal in adults), becoming oblique only after the age of 5. Healthy tonsils in infants and young children may become enlarged, contributing to airway obstruction.

Difficulty in hearing is a crucial symptom that needs to be diagnosed and evaluated without delay. The first two years of life are very important because language development occurs rapidly, with vocabulary being stored in the mind for use in the future. The sense of hearing is crucial to this. Should hearing impairment detrimentally impact on the development of these stores, this level of plasticity does not occur again for such learning in the future. This can clinically present with speech problems in the child, e.g. speech delay.

5.3.3 Presenting symptoms of ENT disease in pediatrics

Ear	Reduced hearing / hearing loss
	Ear pain / pulling the ear / inconsolable crying
	Ear discharge
	Fever
	Tinnitus
	Dizziness
Nose	Mouth breathing
	Rhinorrhea
	Nasal obstruction
	Headache
Throat	Pain in the throat or on swallowing
	Reduced oral intake
	Stridor

5.3.4 Key questions for an ENT history in pediatrics

Take a history using the standard clinical history protocol and **GABDeS** acronym (as per *Section 5.3.1*). In addition, there are a few questions which should be asked, to identify the extent and impact of ear / nasal / sinus or pharyngeal disease on the patient.

In the **general history** be sure to ask about sleep. Due to the relatively small size of the nasal passage, even a small amount of inflammation can obstruct the nose, leading to mouth breathing, snoring, and impaired sleep; this can have a detrimental impact on quality of life and growth of the child.

It is important to elicit if there is a history of **allergy** (to insects, dust mites, pollen, or foods) and atopic conditions, as these can present with rhinitis and asthma and may require lifestyle modifications to see a significant improvement.

Birth history is very important in the neonate and infant patients; ask about any post-natal respiratory difficulties, e.g. needing respiratory support or nebulizers, history of intubation, etc. This may put patients at an increased risk of acute deterioration.

In the **developmental** history, be sure to ask about achievement milestones; recurrent ear infections causing reduced hearing can impact on the development and commencement of speech, which needs urgent and prompt action.

Second-hand smoke causes significant respiratory distress in children; this should be directly asked about in the **social** history. It is also prudent to ask about sick contacts, as infectious diseases are common in childhood.

5.4 Rhinitis

This is inflammation of the nasal lining. Its symptomatology to management are detailed in *Section 3.3*.

In this section we will discuss the key points of this disease relevant to pediatrics; this is not to replace the information in *Section 3.3*.

5.4.1 Causes

In children, common triggers are infection, allergy and environmental factors, e.g. cold weather, cold air / wind.

Its differentials include enlarged adenoids, choanal atresia, and stenosis as causes of nasal obstruction.

5.4.2 Investigation

There are no specific tests advised, as the diagnosis of rhinitis is based on a detailed history and clinical examination. Otolaryngologists may need to perform nasopharyngoscopy. Its cause can be investigated (see details in *Section 3.3*).

If suspected, choanal atresia or stenosis will need radiological investigation via a CT scan of the mid-facial skeleton; this should be requested by pediatric ENT specialists in conjunction with the patient.

5.4.3 Management

The principles of treatment remain the same as in *Section 3.3*; children normally respond well to using hygiene (sea- / salt water) nasal sprays on a regular basis and avoiding relevant allergen exposure. However, it may be difficult for children to tolerate this treatment. There are over the counter saline products designed for little noses.

Steroid nasal spray can lead to growth retardation in young children; however, they are generally considered safe after the age of 2. Thus, children are advised steroid-based nasal spray according to their age, and for a recommended length of time. In the long term these children should have regular growth assessment while on this medication.

Antihistamines (preferably non-sedating) are recommended for mild pediatric rhinitis, with symptoms related to histamine response (sneezing, rhinorrhea, and itching of the nose, palate, and eyes).

5.5 Sinusitis

5.5.1 Introduction

This is inflammation of the lining of the air-filled sinuses in the head. It is almost always associated with rhinitis, hence the term rhinosinusitis is more appropriate. Its symptomatology to management are detailed in *Section 3.5*.

In this section, we will discuss the key points of this disease relevant to pediatrics; this is not to replace the information in *Section 3.5*.

5.5.2 Differential diagnoses

In infants or young children a headache may have many etiologies including eye strain or the need for glasses, as opposed to sinusitis, due to the lack of development of the sinuses in young children.

5.5.3 Diagnosis

Children may present as per *Section 3.5*. However, note that children may present with the less specific symptoms of mouth breathing, irritability, high fever, or periorbital edema. Some may present with OM, with or without effusion.

5.5.4 Management

In most patients, sinusitis usually responds to basic conservative management including saline drops or, if needed, steroid nasal spray or antibiotics. In older children sinusitis is usually more severe as they may not be able to clear out their sinuses regularly or effectively enough.

Immunocompromised children or those with an underlying disease, such as cystic fibrosis, primary ciliary dyskinesia, and immunoglobulin disease, may not respond to such basic conservative management. Those who are not responding need urgent assessment to check for complications and any deterioration, and may even need hospital review. They may require intravenous antibiotic therapy and, in some cases, surgical drainage of the sinuses.

5.5.5 Complications

Although rare, complications are significant and patients should be closely monitored for these including:
- orbital cellulitis
- osteomyelitis of the surrounding bones, meningitis, abscesses (e.g. extradural, sub-dural, or intracranial).

5.5.6 Essential facts

In children with bruising to the eye or extradural hematoma with no history of trauma, sinusitis must be excluded as a cause.

Sinuses are not fully developed at birth; all sinuses develop fully around 8–10 years of age.

5.6 Epistaxis

This is bleeding from the nasal cavity. A guide to assessing this condition can be found in *Section 3.4*.

In this section, we will discuss the key points of this disease relevant to pediatrics; this is not to replace the information in *Section 3.4*.

5.6.1 Introduction

Nosebleeds in children are generally short-lived and self-limiting, although the psychological impact on the child and the concern of parents may be significant. Any child with recurrent nosebleeds should be seen by an ENT specialist.

Epistaxis is not common in those under 2 years old; the peak age is 3–8 years.

5.6.2 Causes

The most common causes of epistaxis in children are:

Most common	Digital trauma (common in children of all ages)
	Lack of humidity / dry environment
	Upper respiratory tract infection (viral or bacterial)
	Foreign body in the nose
Least common	Rarer causes: nasal fracture, blood dyscrasias, nasopharyngeal fibroma, granulomatosis with polyangiitis

If there is an acute nosebleed, immediate action should be in managing the symptom. Once stable, it is important to be brief and precise with your questions when identifying the cause of the nosebleed. The focused history should check for frequency and severity of nosebleeds, and establish the underlying cause from the above common causes.

5.6.3 Management

First aid management of nosebleeds should be commenced in cases of active nosebleed; see *Section 3.4.5*. In short: pinch the nose bilaterally at the anterior tip of the nose (this should be done by the patient / parent / carer) for 10 minutes. Then administer OTC vasoconstrictor. Advise the child to breathe through their mouth, sit up straight and stop whatever they are doing. If needed, plain water mouthwash is advised.

Children with nosebleeds need to be referred to ENT for expert management, as soon as they are seen in primary care clinic. On examination, in very few patients a source of bleeding is recognized.

Once the bleeding has stopped, an ENT specialist should, very carefully, look inside the nose to see if there are any clots. If present they should be removed. If the bleeding vessel is in view then it may be possible to cauterize this; see *Section 3.4.5.*

It is advisable to do this in ENT due to the risk of further trauma, septal perforation, and adhesions. In children with an obvious bleeding point, cautery may be performed with topical lidocaine anesthesia. In case of severe nosebleed, the patient may need nasal packing for a few hours.

5.6.4 Essential facts

On the anterior part of the nasal septum there is a collection of blood vessels called Kiesselbach's plexus, also known as Little's area; this is a common site of nosebleed in all patients.

The nasal mucosa at this very end of the nasal septum is exposed to the environment and is relatively thin; hence the effects of changing temperature, turbulent airflow, and even mild trauma can cause a nosebleed.

5.7 Nasal trauma

5.7.1 Introduction

The nasal structure in children is different to adults, in that the nose is less projected from the facial plane. Secondly, soft tissue and cartilage are sufficiently pliant to allow considerable deformation without permanent injury.

5.7.2 Diagnosis

This history often indicates the cause; if the child is too young to vocalize this there may be history from a parent or other caretaker of sudden onset of symptoms, perhaps within seconds. The patient may present with nosebleed, pain in the nose, facial swelling, blocked nose, or external nasal deformity.

5.7.3 Investigations

Investigations have no significant role as diagnosis is based on history and clinical assessment.

5.7.4 Management

Should the injury cause a fracture, it is usually a greenstick fracture. The swelling usually decreases within 4–5 days, with any minor external nasal deformity significantly improving as the face continues to grow.

Acute, severe deformity affecting functioning of the nose can be corrected under general anesthetic. If the deformity does not improve by the age of 16–18, septoplasty or septorhinoplasty can be performed to correct the nasal septum and improve external nasal deformity.

5.7.5 Complications

The most significant risk after nasal trauma is septal hematoma or abscess. If not treated on time, this could lead to external nasal deformity of a saddle-shaped nose.

5.8 Obstructive sleep apnea

5.8.1 Introduction

Apnea is the absence of breath for at least two attempted breaths. Obstructive sleep apnea (OSA) is when there is a reduction or cessation of oronasal air flow despite continuous thoracic or abdominal respiratory efforts; this cessation can last from 5 to 30 seconds. Its prevalence is 1–5%, most commonly in boys aged 2–5, but it is certainly also seen in older children.

5.8.2 Diagnosis

Children are normally brought in due to loud snoring (and sometimes mouth breathing) often associated with the symptoms and signs of inadequate sleep. Night arousal is very common; the patient may be tossing and turning at night, may wake up tired and have daytime somnolence. They may have behavioral issues including irritability and difficulty concentrating, and may be hyperactive or less active than their peers.

Some children even show signs of decreased weight (failure to thrive). Chronic OSA may give rise to hypoplasia of the mid-face (adenoid facies).

In terms of risk factors, the key one is a preterm birth.

5.8.3 Causes

The most common causes are enlarged tonsils and/or adenoids, rhinitis, and septal deviation (though the latter are comparatively less common). Other causes include structural abnormalities (e.g. macroglossia or retrognathia – which may be part of a genetic syndrome or congenital), Down syndrome, sickle cell disease or cerebral palsy.

OSA should be differentiated from laryngomalacia in infants; in OSA the pitch of the snoring sound is low, compared to the stridor of laryngomalacia.

5.8.4 Investigations

The diagnosis of OSA is made on detailed clinical history and examination. However, definitive diagnosis is made via an overnight sleep study in a sleep lab with pediatric capabilities which will determine the extent of the apnea. A sleep study involves the measurement of multiple physiological variables during sleep, including oxygen saturations, volume of oronasal airway, frequency of airway impairment, spirometry volumes, flow rates, and measurement of end tidal CO_2 to assess for alveolar hypoventilation. The patient's ECG, blood pressure and EEG results are also obtained. This is all brought together and reviewed by a specialist for the purpose of confirming the diagnosis and discussing management. In children, this is a complex test and difficult to perform and if there are complex co-morbidities involved it can be almost impossible.

Sometimes parents record their child's breathing and apneic episodes on their cell phone at initial presentation. This may be helpful although it does not override the need for a good history and examination.

5.8.5 Management

These children should be referred to and managed by a pediatric sleep specialist or otolaryngologist.

Treatment is as directed by the cause: adenotonsillectomy if tonsils and adenoids are enlarged; if rhinitis is present, treat as per *Section 5.4.3*. If structural abnormalities are the root cause, then this will need a discussion between the specialist, patient, and parents.

5.8.6 Essential facts

Mechanism

Oropharyngeal airway patency is maintained by muscle tone. During sleep, pharyngeal structures become relaxed or flaccid, causing some subclinical airway narrowing. Any narrowing of the oropharynx exacerbates the above reduction in air flow. The continuous respiratory efforts give rise to cyclical vibrations of the pharyngeal walls, leading to the production of sounds, i.e. snoring. Note that between each snore is a hypopnea; in severe cases this may lead to true apneic episodes and cessation of pharyngeal airflow.

5.9 Adenoiditis

5.9.1 Introduction

The adenoids are a collection of lymphoid tissue at the back of the nose in the nasopharynx; see *Figure 5.1*. This collection of lymphoid tissue can grow in some children, due to repeated infections.

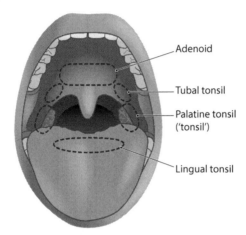

Figure 5.1 Lymphoid ring in the oral cavity.

5.9.2 Diagnosis

Symptomatology arises when the adenoids become infected or enlarged (which is usually due to recurrent infections). The patient may suffer from repeated upper respiratory tract infections, nasal obstruction, epistaxis, or otitis media. On examination, there may be signs of serous OM (see *Section 2.7*).

When adenoids are enlarged, patients may snore or, in some cases, develop OSA (see *Section 5.8*).

5.9.3 Investigations

A detailed history and clinical examination are considered the best diagnostic tools and these aid the decision regarding an adenoidectomy; however, lateral X-ray of the neck can be helpful.

5.9.4 Management

The definitive treatment is adenoidectomy in those who are symptomatic, e.g. suffering recurrent ear infections, constant nasal symptoms due to enlarged adenoids, OSA, or breathing difficulties.

5.10 Cystic fibrosis

5.10.1 Introduction

Cystic fibrosis is an autosomal recessive inherited condition which affects the exocrine glands (incidence 1 in 3400 in the US). As such, it has an impact on the respiratory (both lower and upper tract), hepatobiliary, and fertility systems.

5.10.2 Diagnosis

This usually presents in early life via a positive newborn blood spot screening test or, less commonly, symptomatology. Diagnoses are usually made by the age of 2 years, although some cases are diagnosed in adulthood.

Patients may present symptoms of ENT disease: recurring respiratory tract infections, shortness of breath, persistent cough, recurrent sinus infections, nasal polyps (a RED FLAG in children), recurrent ear infections and effusions. Generally, there is difficulty gaining weight and diarrhea.

5.10.3 Investigations

As mentioned above, there is a screening test: the newborn blood spot test. The diagnosis is then made on a sweat test and genetic testing for the anomaly on the *CFTR* gene.

5.10.4 Management

Unfortunately, there is no cure yet for cystic fibrosis; however, patients are living longer due to early diagnosis and better treatments. Patients should be managed by pediatrics and pediatric specialty teams. Treatment is designed to provide symptomatic relief in order to improve patients' quality of life and avoid complications.

In terms of ENT symptoms, there are mucus-thinning medications, physical therapy to help remove thick secretions via postural drainage, and antibiotics for infection.

Patients should also receive anti-inflammatory medication, bronchodilators, medicine to replace pancreatic enzymes, and multivitamins.

5.10.5 Complications

Later in life patients may develop chronic respiratory failure, diabetes mellitus, malnutrition, infertility, and osteoporosis, among other disorders.

5.11 Hearing loss and deafness

Deafness is the inability to hear and understand sounds. A guide to assessing this condition can be found in *Section 2.3*.

In this section, we will discuss the key points of this disease relevant to pediatrics; this is not to replace the information in *Section 2.3*.

5.11.1 Introduction

Depending upon their age, young people (especially infants and young children) may not be able to vocalize their inability to hear. Thus, surrogate markers should be used to recognize the consequences of this inability; for example, a patient fails to respond via eye or head movement when sounds are made outside of their visual field, there is a lack of facial expression in response to conversation, they turn their head away or are distracted when in a conversation, or their speech is delayed or they respond with inappropriate words.

They may lack the ability to build their vocabulary, show poor language development and repeat the same words, at an age where this would not be expected; these may all be hallmarks of a child who cannot hear or has significantly reduced hearing.

5.11.2 Causes

These have been extensively discussed in *Section 2.3*; however, in pediatrics the most common causes include:
- wax in the external auditory canal
- foreign body in the ear
- adenoiditis
- serous OM
- congenital hearing loss.

5.11.3 Investigations

The hearing assessment should be carried out as per *Section 2.3*; however, there will be some variation relevant to children.

The newborn hearing screening program is performed in the antenatal period before the infant leaves the hospital, to help identify moderate–profound deafness or hearing impairment, with referral to specialist care if the neonate fails the screening test. **Otoacoustic emissions** (OAE) and **auditory brainstem response** (ABR) may help evaluate hearing in young children. These are generally ordered at the specialist level.

Play audiometry is where behavioral audiometric testing is done in a soundproof room. The child is shown how to perform a repetitive play task, such as placing a peg on a keyboard each time they hear a sound.
- The *normal* range for hearing is 10–20 decibels (dB) and 500–4000 Hertz (Hz).

- *Mild* hearing loss is 21–40 dB, *moderate* is 41–70 dB, *severe* is 71–95 dB, while *profound* deafness is >95 dB.

In older children, a routine audiogram can be performed.

Tympanometry (see *Section 1.5.2*) is a valuable component of the audiometric evaluation. It is an objective examination used to test the function of the middle ear through mobility of the tympanic membrane and middle ear bones by creating variation of air pressure in the ear canal. In infants, this is usually the only test that is done to identify a conduction defect in an outpatient clinic.

Other objective tests, for example central auditory processing, can be advised in severe cases but are usually requested by specialists (see *Sections 1.5.4* and *1.5.5*).

5.11.4 Management

This is used on the identified cause; see *Section 2.2*. In short, this may encompass removal of ear wax, PE tubes for serous OM, removal of a foreign body from the ear, or adenoidectomy for recurrent adenoiditis.

If there is no treatable cause, the child should be referred to pediatric audiology for specialty evaluation and for consultation with specialists and the provision of a hearing aid. There may be a speech deficit in children with hearing loss. Local school districts are required to provide speech pathology services for children aged 3 and older with speech deficits. Younger children may receive community services which vary by location, and school-age children may receive evaluation for a possible Individual Educational Plan (IEP) through their schools based on disability. These children should be followed up regularly long-term, to monitor and support the development of their speech and the progress of their hearing.

5.12 Acute otitis media

This is an infection of the middle ear space; see *Figure 2.1*. Its symptomatology through to management are detailed in *Section 2.7*.

In this section, we will discuss the key points of this disease relevant to pediatrics; this is not to replace the information in *Section 2.7*.

5.12.1 Introduction

This is the most common cause of hearing loss in childhood with a prevalence of 20% in the 2–7 years age group.

5.12.2 Investigations

Tympanogram (see *Section 1.5.2*) and audiogram (see *Section 1.5.1*), or play audiogram (see *Section 5.11.3*) may be requested to identify the presence of an effusion or to determine the nature and extent of hearing loss, respectively.

5.12.3 Management

See *Section 2.7.4*. The majority of cases will resolve spontaneously within three months; however, the patient should be monitored for the development of complications.

Children 2 years of age and older are usually treated with inhaled nasal steroid sprays. Effusions that fail to clear within 3 months are generally taken to the operating room for myringotomy and pressure equalizing tube insertion (BMT). This allows for equalization of pressures in the middle ear.

5.12.4 Complications

- Mastoiditis – see *Section 2.7.5*.
- Serous OM – this can be due to Eustachian tube dysfunction. This is further exacerbated by the fact that the tube is horizontal (only becoming more diagonal, as in adulthood, after the age of 5). This means that infections of the nose find it easier to migrate up to the ear. This can be addressed by myringotomy and tympanostomy (insertion of a ventilation tube into the tympanic membrane), known colloquially as a PE (pressure equalizing) tube.
- Chronic OM – this is when there is recurrent or resistant middle ear infection. If symptoms have not improved in 4–6 weeks it is advised that patients are referred to ENT.

- ○ Sometimes in these cases there is a perforation of the tympanic membrane (sudden onset of yellow or blood-stained discharge), after which acute symptoms improve significantly.
- ○ If a cholesteatoma is suspected (see *Section 2.8*), specialists should consider ordering CT (preferred) or MRI imaging studies to confirm the presence of a cholesteatoma and its extent; when given the time and space to grow, cholesteatomas can be far-reaching.

5.13 Tinnitus

5.13.1 Introduction

Tinnitus is the perception of sound without external stimulation (see *Section 2.18* for additional information). It occurs frequently in adulthood (albeit often intermittently) and some children (even as young as 4 years) may also complain of hearing 'noises' in their ear e.g. buzzing, ringing, or, in some cases, music.

It is estimated to affect up to 29% of children.

5.13.2 Causes

Please see *Section 2.2*. The key diagnoses in children are:
- ear infection
- loud noise exposure, especially the use of ear-/headphones
- head injury
- foreign body in the ear
- medication-induced, e.g. chemotherapy
- idiopathic.

It should be noted that patients may perceive that the sound, irrespective of cause, becomes worse when they are anxious.

5.13.3 Investigations

A tympanogram (see *Section 1.5.2*), which looks for signs of an effusion in the middle ear, and an audiogram (see *Section 1.5.1*), which looks for any hearing loss and the nature of this, may be requested if such a diagnosis is being considered.

5.13.4 Management

The impact on a child's quality of life due to this symptom should not be underestimated; it can also have a marked effect on sleep.

After ruling out dangerous causes, reassurance is needed as well as management techniques. The latter can be done in pediatric audiology, which will also provide long-term management advice and follow-up.

Explaining this symptom to a young child may be a difficult task; patience along with a patient-guided and patient-centered approach is needed by the clinician. Indeed, children are often quite inquisitive, even more so than adults at times, and often discuss how the condition and their symptoms co-relate with one another. These children need lots of support. In a very few cases, children may respond well to a white noise generator.

5.14 Vertigo

5.14.1 Introduction

Vertigo is the sensation of rotation without stimulus.

5.14.2 Diagnosis

It is important to be clear about the symptoms; does the child describe a rotatory sensation or are they describing the sensation of light-headedness? Does the child feel they are spinning or the room is spinning around them? Children suffering from this are usually fearful and want to remain close to their parents; in such cases, patience and cooperation with the child is key.

During episodes, the child may vomit and complain of feeling generally unwell. Associated symptoms, as below, will be key to the history.

5.14.3 Causes

The table below shows the causes of vertigo, together with symptom cluster and signs (bear in mind that not all may be present).

Migraine	Headache, usually bilateral (may later become lateralized), GI upset, visual disturbance which may occur with vertigo more than headache
Infection of inner ear e.g. secondary to a cholesteatoma	Fever, tinnitus, hearing loss, or reduced hearing On examination: a discharging ear and cholesteatoma may be visualized
Seizures	History of seizure / previous similar episode, urinary or bowel incontinence, tongue biting
Head injury or whiplash injury	History of incident injury, headache, swelling on head, bony tenderness
Ophthalmic disorders	Visual disturbance, strabismus

5.14.4 Investigations

These should be directed as per the working diagnosis and would include an audiogram (see *Section 1.5.1*) to assess the extent and nature of hearing loss, a tympanogram (see *Section 1.5.2*) to assess for hearing loss and presence of an effusion. A caloric test (see *Section 1.6.1*) can be requested in older children; this is used to assess vestibular function. Other extensive vestibular function tests and a CT scan of petrous temporal bone (looking for cholesteatoma or any other mass lesion) may also be performed.

5.14.5 Management

Any child complaining of dizziness, with no clear alternative non-ENT diagnoses, should be referred to ENT for careful evaluation of vestibular dysfunction. The treatment is directed to the cause, e.g. treatment for migrainous attack with prophylaxis (if needed).

For vestibular dysfunction, vestibular rehabilitation should be carried out by a physical therapist and audiologist as soon as possible following a diagnosis of vertigo. Medical treatment is not recommended first-line but could be used in acutely symptomatic patients. These children need a lot of support with regular follow-up.

5.15 Laryngeal papillomatosis

5.15.1 Introduction

This is a benign non-cancerous growth on the larynx, usually presenting in those aged 2–3 years.

5.15.2 Diagnosis

Laryngeal papillomatosis commonly presents with voice change; there may be a croaky quality to the voice, a weak cry, or abnormalities in voice volume and tone. There may be respiratory complications, e.g. chronic cough and noisy breathing. Some parents also note that there is associated poor feeding. Basic bedside clinical examination does not usually elicit any specific symptoms but is used to exclude other diagnoses.

5.15.3 Causes

This is caused by the human papillomavirus (types 6 and 11 have been implicated).

5.15.4 Investigations

In ENT, pediatric nasopharyngoscopy may be performed. However, direct laryngoscopy under general anesthetic is the procedure of choice; the lesion can be directly visualized, removed, and a sample sent for histology. This is known as microlaryngoscopy with excision and biopsy.

5.15.5 Management

See *Section 5.15.4*. The growth may reoccur and affected children may require multiple microlaryngoscopies with excision of growth in their lifetime.

Chapter 6

Systemic disease affecting ears, nose, and throat

6.1	Introduction	154
6.2	Skin disorders	154
6.3	Eye	154
6.4	Nervous system and neurological diseases	155
6.5	Endocrine diseases	155
6.6	Congenital disorders	155
6.7	Vascular disease	155
6.8	Maxillofacial diseases	156
6.9	Bone and joint pathology	156
6.10	Gastroenterology	156
6.11	Medication	156

6.1 Introduction

Throughout this book we have discussed how abnormalities in the anatomy and/or physiology of the ear, nose, and throat as independent organs can lead to disease. In this chapter, we will look at clinically prevalent diseases affecting other body systems and how they can affect ears, noses, and throats.

6.2 Skin disorders

The external ear and external auditory canal are particularly sensitive to such conditions.

- **Eczema** can affect the skin of the pinna, external auditory meatus, and canal, which may lead to **recurrent otitis media**.
- **Psoriasis** can involve the pinna and external auditory canal, which can cause **otitis externa**.
- **Skin cancer** can affect the **pinna** and skin of the **nose**, as they are in positions where they can be significantly exposed to sunshine.
- **Herpes simplex infections** can involve any nerve root in the body; when infecting the facial ganglion they can cause **painful vesicles on the pinna, external auditory canal**, and parts of the face.
- **Fungal skin infections** can involve the external auditory canal, leading to **fungal otitis externa** (also known as otomycosis). Fungal infection can also involve the sinuses.
- **Seborrhea** of the scalp may also cause **seborrheic otitis externa**.

6.3 Eye diseases

The nose and eye are directly linked via the nasolacrimal duct and as such, are susceptible to diseases affecting the other.

- **Injury** to the *ethmoid* sinus can involve the orbital plate and lamina papyracea, and trauma to the *maxillary* sinus may involve the floor of the orbit.
- **Sinusitis** of the *ethmoid* sinus, in particular, may involve orbital contents if there is dehiscence of the orbital plate / lamina papyracea, and can lead to **orbital cellulitis**. Sinusitis involving the *sphenoid* sinus can lead to a **visual defect**. Sinusitis affecting the *frontal* sinus can also involve the **orbit**.
- **Nasal polypectomy** and antral washout may cause damage to the lamina papyracea and floor of the orbit, which can lead to **orbital cellulitis** and, in severe cases, **cavernous sinus thrombosis**.
- **Cancer** of the nasopharynx can cause abducens (6th cranial nerve) nerve palsy which supplies the lateral rectus muscle of the eye. This may present as convergent strabismus.

6.4 Nervous system and neurological diseases

Due to the complex functions of the organs of the ENT, neurological abnormality can significantly impact on their ability to function normally.

- **Referred pain:** cancer of the tongue can present with deep-seated **earache**.
- **Mastoiditis** can present as **facial weakness** / paralysis by impairing the function of the facial nerve (7th cranial nerve).
- **Trigeminal neuralgia** can present with **mid-facial pain** and **earache**.
- **Glossopharyngeal neuralgia** can present with deep-seated **earache**.
- **Multiple sclerosis** can cause **dizziness**, hoarseness of voice, and **dysphagia**, due to the involvement of the nerves supplying the organs.

6.5 Endocrine diseases

- **Hypothyroidism** can present with **rhinitis** symptoms, **change in voice**, and **fatigue**.
- **Goiter** can present with pressure symptoms including **dysphagia**, **change in voice**, and **choking sensation**, particularly when lying down.
- **Diabetes** can present with **recurrent furuncles in the ear** or **recurrent otitis externa**.
- **Pregnancy** can cause **rhinitis**.

6.6 Congenital disorders

There are many congenitally inherited syndromes, such as **Down syndrome**, which can cause **hearing impairment** of the infant.

- **Cleft palate** can cause **serous OM**, leading to **reduced hearing**. It may present as a **change in voice** or at the neonatal examination.
- **Ectodermal dysplasia** can present as **glue ear** and **recurrent rhinosinusitis**.
- **Osler–Rendu–Weber disease** may present with **epistaxis** and **hemorrhagic spots** on the **tongue**.
- **Congenital cholesteatoma** may present later in life; see *Section 2.8*.
- **Laryngomalacia** of the soft cartilages of the larynx can impact on breathing, causing **stridor** and, in severe cases, respiratory distress and **difficulties in feeding** of the infant.
- **Preauricular sinus** can present with **recurrent infection**.
- **Branchial cyst** can present as a **neck lump**.

6.7 Vascular disease

ENT organs have an extensive blood supply and as such are susceptible to lesions of this nature.

- **Bleeding disorders** can lead to **epistaxis**.
- **Vascular abnormality** of the inner head can cause **tinnitus**.
- **Raised blood pressure or hypertension** can present as **epistaxis** and **dizziness**.
- **Anemia** can present with an **off-balance** feeling, **dizziness**, and **dysphagia**.
- **Glomus jugulare tumors** can present as **tinnitus** and **hearing loss** on the affected side.

6.8 Maxillofacial diseases

The ear and sinuses are in close proximity to structural bones of the face and head.

- **Temporomandibular joint** arthralgia can present as deep-seated earache on the affected side.
- **Maxillary sinusitis** can present as **incisor teeth numbness** and maxillary tooth pain.
- **Dental cancer** can present as recurrent maxillary **sinusitis** and oroantral **fistula**.

6.9 Bone and joint pathology

- **Arthritis** of the neck bones can lead to an **off-balance** feeling and **tinnitus.**
- **Fracture of the maxilla** involving the floor of the orbit can cause sagging of the eye on the affected side.
- **Cervical spondylitis** can cause **dizziness** and **dysphagia** due to prominent osteophytes.

6.10 Gastroenterology

The below diseases of the GI system can cause symptoms of the nose and throat.

- **Hyperacidity** can lead to **hoarseness** of voice and **sensation of a foreign body** in the throat. It can also lead to excessive **post-nasal discharge**.
- **Acid reflux** in children can lead to **middle ear infection**.

On the other hand, there are ENT diseases which can also present with GI symptoms.

- **Post-nasal discharge** in acute and acute-on-chronic rhinosinusitis or severe rhinitis can lead to hyperacidity.

6.11 Medication

Many commonly prescribed medications can cause symptoms of the ENT.

- **Beta-blockers** can cause **nasal obstruction** and **rhinitis**.
- **ACE inhibitors** can cause a dry **cough**.
- **Hormone replacement therapy** patients (and those going through puberty or menopause, due to hormonal changes) may suffer from **rhinitis**.
- **Erythromycin, vancomycin, neomycin, and chemotherapy treatment** can lead to **tinnitus** or make tinnitus worse.
- **Frusemide and ethacrynic acid**, and **aspirin** and other **NSAIDs** can cause **tinnitus** or make it worse.
- **Aspirin sensitivity** can cause **rhinitis**, **nasal polyp**, and **asthma**.

Chapter 7
Key operations in ENT

This chapter is designed to give you the gist of some of the most common ENT procedures. It will not cover everything and is not in enough detail to suffice as a consent form. The patient will need to ask their doctor about specific issues, e.g. taking time off school / work, ability to drive, medications to be discharged on, and any follow-up appointment.

Patients should discuss any surgical concerns with their otolaryngology specialist / ENT surgeon.

	Tonsillectomy	Adenoidectomy	Septorhinoplasty
Summary of the procedure	To surgically remove the palatine tonsils from the throat. The patient is under a general anesthetic.	To surgically remove the adenoids from the back of the nose. The patient is under a general anesthetic.	To surgically straighten the nasal septum and correct any external nasal deformity. The patient is under a general anesthetic.
Pre-operative preparation by the patient*	Nothing by mouth 6 hours prior to the operation. Tell the doctor if the patient has an acute infection of ear, nose, or throat in the days before the procedure.	Nothing by mouth 6 hours prior to the operation. Tell the doctor if the patient has an acute infection of ear, nose, or throat in the days before the procedure.	Nothing by mouth 6 hours prior to the operation. Tell the doctor if the patient has an acute infection of ear, nose, or throat in the days before the procedure.
Approx. duration of op	30–45 minutes	15 minutes	60 minutes
Admission type	Outpatient surgery, home same day	Outpatient surgery, home same day	Usually outpatient surgery, home same day (or within 24 hours)
Signs to look out for – to contact a doctor urgently⁺	Spitting out or vomiting blood / clots – **GO TO ED** (*a bit of blood-stained spit on 1ˢᵗ day is expected*). Severe pain in the throat or ear. Not being able to eat or drink / being dehydrated.	Bleeding (via nose or mouth) – **GO TO ED**. Severe pain. Not being able to eat or drink / being dehydrated.	Nosebleed – **GO TO ED** (*some dark bloodstained discharge may occur on 1ˢᵗ day*). Difficulty breathing / worsening of nasal blockage – **GO TO ED** (*for 1ˢᵗ week you may feel stuffiness of the nose*). Severe pain.

*This is generic advice which does not replace advice patients are given by their healthcare professional. Make sure they attend their pre-assessment clinic appointment – be sure they mention any dental work they may have, e.g. loose teeth / caps. Please discuss any medication they are on before their operation with a doctor to find out if they need to stop any of them before the operation – it is especially important to discuss blood-thinning medication. Emphasize the importance of stopping smoking before their operation and support the patient's attempt to quit (smoking can impact recovery time and increase the risk of developing blood clots). The patient should be made aware that they should arrange for someone to take them home.

Functional endoscopic sinus surgery (FESS)	Nasal polypectomy	PE tube insertion	Mastoid exploration
To aid clearance of infection or blockage of the sinuses and remove any nasal polyps. The patient is under a general anesthetic.	To surgically remove polyps from the nose. The patient is under a general anesthetic.	Also known as myringotomy, with ventilation tube insertion placed into the eardrum. The patient is under a general anesthetic.	To surgically clear disease from mastoid cavity and middle ear. The patient is under a general anesthetic.
Nothing by mouth 6 hours prior to the operation. Tell the doctor if the patient has an acute infection of ear, nose, or throat in the days before the procedure.	Nothing by mouth 6 hours prior to the operation. Tell the doctor if the patient has an acute infection of ear, nose, or throat in the days before the procedure.	To have had a hearing test beforehand. Nothing by mouth 6 hours prior to the operation.	To have had a hearing test beforehand. Nothing by mouth 6 hours prior to the operation. Tell the doctor if the patient has an acute infection of ear, nose, or throat in the days before the procedure.
60 minutes	45 minutes	15 minutes	45 minutes
Outpatient surgery, home same day	Outpatient surgery, home same day	Outpatient surgery, home same day	Inpatient (approx. 24 hours)
Nosebleed – **GO TO ED** (*dried blood is expected, especially on 1ˢᵗ day*). Difficulty breathing / worsening of nasal blockage – **GO TO ED** (*for 1ˢᵗ week you may feel stuffiness of the nose*). Severe pain. Tenderness over sinuses or foul-tasting post-nasal drip.	Nosebleed – **GO TO ED** (*dried blood is expected, especially on 1ˢᵗ day*). Tenderness over sinuses or foul-tasting post-nasal drip.	Ear discharge / dizziness / bleeding. Pain in the ear.	Off-balance dizziness. Ear discharge.

⁺This should not replace clinical assessment / concern. This does not encompass all the complications and side-effects of an operation; it simply shows some key signs the patient should look out for. It also does not detail any immediate post-operative interventions that the patient may have or need, e.g. the nose may be packed after nasal surgery.

Index

Bold indicates main entry

Achalasia, 98, **102**
Acoustic neuroma, 17, 23, 27, 28, **43**, 56, 58
Adenoidectomy, 143, 158
Adenoiditis, **143**, 145
Anaphylaxis, 114, 116
Anatomy
 of the ear, 20
 of the nose, 68
 of the throat, 96
Anosmia, 71, **85**
Aphthous ulcer, *see* Ulcer
Audiogram
 play audiometry, **145**
 pure tone, **10**
 speech, **13**

Bell's palsy, 24, **61–2**
Benign paroxysmal positional vertigo (BPPV), **51**
Beta transferrin test, 84
Bone and joint pathology affecting ears, nose, and throat, 156

Caloric test, **15**, 56
Cerumen, *see* Wax
Change in voice, 98, **109**, 112, 155
Cholesteatoma, **23–4**, 33, 35, 53
 acquired, **36**
 congenital, **36**, 155
Ciprofloxacin, 66

Congenital disorders affecting ears, nose, and throat, 155
Croup, 116, **119**
Cystic fibrosis, 73, **144**

Differential diagnoses
 of ear problems, 23
 of nose problems, 71
 of throat problems, 98
Dix–Hallpike test, 51
Dizziness, 15, 24, **49**, 53, 56, 59, 151
Dysphagia, 98, **100**, 102

Earache, **47**, 65, 155, 156
Ear discharge, 4, 17, 23, 36, 38, **45**, 62, 133
Eczema, 23, 31, 45, 154
Electronystagmography, **15**, 56
Endocrine diseases affecting ears, nose, and throat, 155
Epiglottitis (acute), **118–19**, 131
Epistaxis, 71, **77**, 138, 155
Epworth scale, 92
Equi test, **16**, 56
Exostosis, 26–7
Eye disorders affecting ears, nose, and throat, 154

Facial paralysis, 24, 35, **61**
Foreign body
 in the ear, 65
 in the nose, 88

sensation of, 156
in the throat, 123
Fracture of the nasal bone,
71, **83**
Functional endoscopic sinus surgery
(FESS), 159
Fungal ear infection, **31**, 154
Furuncle
in the ear, 23, 45, **66**
in the nose, 89

Gastroenterology disorders affecting ears,
nose and throat, 156
Globus pharyngeus, 98, **102**
Glomus tumor, 26
Glucose test (for diabetes), 32, **44**, 84, 89, 155

Halitosis, 99, **124**
Hearing loss
in children, 145
conductive, 25
post-surgery, 42
sensorineural, 25
sudden onset, 28
Hereditary angioneurotic edema, **117**
Hydrocortisone, 66

Imbalance, 49

Kiesselbach's plexus, 139

Labyrinthitis, 24, 35, 49, 51
Lacrimation
loss of, 63
test, 63
Laryngeal papillomatosis, 109, **152**
Laryngitis, 112

Malignant otitis externa, 26, **32**, 62
Mastoid
cavity, 35
exploration, 159
process, **4**, 8
Mastoiditis, 23, 25, **35**, 155
Maxillofacial diseases affecting ears,
nose, and throat, 156
Medication affecting ears, nose, and
throat, 156
Ménière's disease, 23–4, 49, **55**

Nasal polypectomy, 154, **159**
Nasal spray, 75–6
Nasal trauma, 140
Neck
lump, 6, 99, **126**, 155
triangles (anterior and posterior), 126
Neurological diseases affecting ears,
nose, and throat, 155

Obstructive sleep apnea, **92**, 141
Olfactory area, 68–9
Ossicles, 12, **21**
Osteoma, 26, **27**
Otitis externa, 23, 26, **31**, 154
Otitis media
acute, **33–4**, 147
chronic suppurative, 23, 26, **33–4**
serous, **33–4**, 58, 62, 145, 147, 155
Otosclerosis, 12, 23, 26, **40–1**, 58
Otoscopy, 4
Otovent nasal balloon, 34

Pediatric ENT history taking, 132
Perforation
septal, 90
tympanic membrane, 23, 26,
35, **38**
Peritonsillar abscess, 98, 104, **106**
PE tube, 34, 63, **147**, 159
insertion of, 159
Pharyngeal pouch, 98, **102**
Pharyngitis, **107–8**
Polyp
nasal, **5–6**, 71, 159
treatment of nasal, 75
vocal cord, **109**, 110, 111
Presbycusis, 23, **59**

Quinsy, see Peritonsillar abscess

Ramsay Hunt syndrome, 23, **62**
Rhinitis, **72**, 135
Rinne test, see Tuning fork test
Romberg test, 55
Round window, 21–2

Salivary gland stones, 99, **121**, 126
Septal abscess, **83**, 84
Septal hematoma, **83**, 84, 140

Septorhinoplasty, 158
Sialogram, **18**, 121, 127
Sinusitis, 71, 72, **80**, 136
Skin disorders affecting ears, nose,
    and throat, 154
Speech therapy, 110
Stridor, 99, **114**, 117–19, 155
Syncope, 49

Temporomandibular joint, 47
Tinnitus, 24, 55, **149**, 155–6
Tonsillectomy, 105, **158**
Tonsillolith, 105
Tuning fork test, 8–9

Ulcer, aphthous, 99, **120**, 124
Unterberg test, 55

Utricle, 22
Uvulopalatopharyngoplasty, **93**, 105

Vascular disease affecting ears, nose,
    and throat, 155
Vertigo, **49**, 150
Vestibular function test, **15**, 55–6

Wax, 20, 23, 25, **30**, 145
Weber and Rinne test, *see* Tuning
    fork test
White noise generator, **59**, 149

X-ray
    lateral neck, 118
    nasal bone, 83
    post-nasal space, 143